Women's Preventive Health Care

Editors

JEANNE A. CONRY
MAUREEN G. PHIPPS

OBSTETRICS AND GYNECOLOGY CLINICS OF NORTH AMERICA

www.obgyn.theclinics.com

Consulting Editor
WILLIAM F. RAYBURN

September 2019 • Volume 46 • Number 3

ELSEVIER

1600 John F. Kennedy Boulevard ● Suite 1800 ● Philadelphia, Pennsylvania, 19103-2899

http://www.theclinics.com

OBSTETRICS AND GYNECOLOGY CLINICS OF NORTH AMERICA Volume 46, Number 3
September 2019 ISSN 0889-8545, ISBN-13: 978-0-323-68351-7

Editor: Kerry Holland
Developmental Editor: Kristen Helm

Obstetrics and Gynecology Clinics (ISSN 0889-8545) is published quarterly by Elsevier Inc., 360 Park Avenue South, New York, NY 10010-1710. Months of issue are March, June, September, and December. Periodicals postage paid at New York, NY, and additional mailing offices. Subscription price per year is $322.00 (US individuals), $685.00 (US institutions), $100.00 (US students), $404.00 (Canadian individuals), $865.00 (Canadian institutions), $225.00 (Canadian students), $459.00 (international individuals), $865.00 (international institutions), and $225.00 (international students). To receive student/resident rate, orders must be accompanied by name of affiliated institution, date of term, and the signature of program/residency coordinator on institution letterhead. Orders will be billed at individual rate until proof of status is received. Foreign air speed delivery is included in all *Clinics* subscription prices. All prices are subject to change without notice. POSTMASTER: Send address changes to *Obstetrics and Gynecology Clinics*, Elsevier Health Sciences Division, Subscription Customer Service, 3251 Riverport Lane, Maryland Heights, MO 63043. **Customer Service: Telephone: 1-800-654-2452 (U.S. and Canada); 314-447-8871 (outside U.S. and Canada). Fax: 314-447-8029. E-mail: journalscustomerservice-usa@elsevier.com (for print support); journalsonlinesupport-usa@elsevier. com (for online support).**

Reprints. For copies of 100 or more of articles in this publication, please contact the Commercial Reprints Department, Elsevier Inc., 360 Park Avenue South, New York, New York 10010-1710. Tel.: 212-633-3874; Fax: 212-633-3820; E-mail: reprints@elsevier.com.

Obstetrics and Gynecology Clinics of North America is also published in Spanish by McGraw-Hill Interamericana Editores S.A., P.O. Box 5-237, 06500, Mexico; in Portuguese by Reichmann and Affonso Editores, Rio de Janeiro, Brazil; and in Greek by Paschalidis Medical Publications, Athens, Greece.

Obstetrics and Gynecology Clinics of North America is covered in MEDLINE/PubMed (Index Medicus), Excerpta Medica, Current Concepts/Clinical Medicine, Science Citation Index, BIOSIS, CINAHL, and ISI/BIOMED.

Contributors

CONSULTING EDITOR

WILLIAM F. RAYBURN, MD, MBA
Associate Dean, Continuing Medical Education and Professional Development, Distinguished Professor and Emeritus Chair, Obstetrics and Gynecology, University of New Mexico School of Medicine, Albuquerque, New Mexico

EDITORS

JEANNE A. CONRY, MD, PhD
Past President, The American College of Obstetricians and Gynecologists, President-elect, The International Federation of Gynecology and Obstetrics, President, The Environmental Health Leadership Foundation, Granite Bay, California

MAUREEN G. PHIPPS, MD, MPH
Chief Executive Officer, The American College of Obstetricians and Gynecologists, Chair and Chace-Joukowsky Professor, Department of Obstetrics and Gynecology, Assistant Dean for Teaching and Research in Women's Health, Warren Alpert Medical School of Brown University, Professor of Epidemiology, Brown University School of Public Health, Chief of Obstetrics and Gynecology, Women and Infants Hospital and Care, New England Health System, Providence, Rhode Island

AUTHORS

PRIYA BATRA, PsyD
Women's Health Psychologist, Kaiser Permanente, Women's Health, Sacramento, California

CAROLYN J. CRANDALL, MD, MS, FACP
Professor of Medicine, David Geffen School of Medicine, University of California, Los Angeles, UCLA Medicine/GIM, Los Angeles, California

MARK S. DeFRANCESCO, MD, MBA, FACOG
Assistant Clinical Professor, Department of Obstetrics and Gynecology, University of Connecticut, Farmington, Connecticut; Chief Medical Officer (Emeritus), Women's Health Connecticut, Avon, Connecticut; Past President, American College of Obstetricians and Gynecologists, Washington, DC

NATHANIEL DeNICOLA, MD, MSHP
Assistant Professor of Obstetrics and Gynecology, The George Washington University, Washington, DC

MEGAN L. EVANS, MD, MPH
Assistant Professor, Department of Obstetrics and Gynecology, Tufts University School of Medicine, Associate Residency Program Director, Tufts Medical Center, Boston, Massachusetts

MEADOW MAZE GOOD, DO, FACOG
Assistant Professor, Chief Female Pelvic Medicine & Reconstructive Surgery, Department of Obstetrics and Gynecology, University of Florida College of Medicine Jacksonville, Jacksonville, Florida

AFSHAN B. HAMEED, MD
Professor of Clinical Obstetrics and Gynecology, Department of Obstetrics and Gynecology, Division of Maternal-Fetal Medicine, Department of Medicine, Division of Cardiology, University of California, Irvine Medical Center, Orange, California

ELIZABETH A. HOOVER, MD
Department of Obstetrics and Gynecology, Division of Maternal Fetal Medicine, University of South Florida, Tampa, Florida

JUDETTE M. LOUIS, MD, MPH
Department of Obstetrics and Gynecology, Division of Maternal Fetal Medicine, University of South Florida, Tampa, Florida

KRISTEN A. MATTESON, MD, MPH
Associate Professor of Obstetrics and Gynecology, Division of Research, Department of Obstetrics and Gynecology, Women and Infants Hospital, Warren Alpert Medical School of Brown University, Providence, Rhode Island

KELLY McCUE, MD
Chief, Obstetrics and Gynecology, The Permanente Medical Group, Sacramento, California

MARY JANE MINKIN, MD, FACOG, NCMP
Clinical Professor, Department of Obstetrics, Gynecology and Reproductive Sciences, Yale University School of Medicine, New Haven, Connecticut

RACHEL A. NEWMAN, MD, MBA
Resident Physician, Department of Obstetrics and Gynecology, University of California, Irvine Medical Center, Orange, California

DIANA E. RAMOS, MD, MPH
Associate Clinical Professor, Department of Obstetrics and Gynecology, Keck University of Southern California, Los Angeles, California

ELLEN R. SOLOMON, MD, FACOG
Assistant Professor, Obstetrics and Gynecology, Division of Female Pelvic Surgery, University of Massachusetts–Baystate Medical Center, Springfield, Massachusetts

NICHOLE A. TYSON, MD
Department of Obstetrics and Gynecology, The Permanente Medical Group, Roseville; Associate Clinical Faculty, UC Davis Medical Center, Sacramento, California

ALISON VOGELL, MD
Assistant Professor, Department of Obstetrics and Gynecology, Tufts University School of Medicine, Residency Program Director, Tufts Medical Center, Boston, Massachusetts

KATE M. ZALUSKI, MD
Assistant Professor of Obstetrics and Gynecology, Clinician Educator, Division of Emergency Obstetrics and Gynecology, Department of Obstetrics and Gynecology, Women and Infants Hospital, Warren Alpert Medical School of Brown University, Providence, Rhode Island

Contents

Section 1 - Reproductive Age

An investment in assuring the health of women, before pregnancy, can reap improved health for women, children, and their families. A paradigm shift of health must occur if perinatal outcomes are to improve, moving beyond reactive care to preventive or preconception care. Preconception health is centered on an assumption a woman is planning on becoming pregnant. But for many women, pregnancy is unplanned and medical conditions may have a negative impact on the trajectory of pregnancy and health. A new paradigm focusing on prevention and wellness can prepare women for lifelong health and healthy perinatal outcomes.

Contraception is paramount to the overall health and longevity of women. Most women in the United States use birth control in their reproductive lifetimes. All options should be available and easily accessible to permit individualization and optimization of chosen methods. Current contraceptive methods available in the United States are reviewed. Emergency contraception, contraception in the postpartum period, and strategies to tailor methods to those affected by partner violence are also addressed. Tables and flow charts help providers and patients compare various contraceptive methods, optimize the start of a method, and identify resources for addressing safety in those with underlying medical conditions.

Pregnancy complications provide insight into women's future health risks and have long term implications for maternal and child health. Obesity has been associated with adverse perinatal outcomes and is a risk factor for chronic disease. Excessive weight gain during pregnancy often translates into postpartum weight retention, increasing women's risk for obesity. Pregnancy and the postpartum period provides a unique opportunity to discuss health beyond pregnancy, emphasize interconception care, and implement appropriate prevention strategies. We aim to review the impact of obesity, gestational weight gain, postpartum weight retention, and role of nutrition and exercise on pregnancy and lifelong health.

Menstrual health assessment facilitates identification of pathologic conditions (eg, abnormal uterine bleeding, endometriosis), offers the opportunity to educate women on what menstrual symptoms may be normal or abnormal, and provides the opportunity to initiate treatment for women who are suffering because of problems with menstrual bleeding or associated symptoms. Heavy bleeding, pain, fatigue, and mood changes significantly affect a woman's physical, social, and emotional quality of life. Promptly identifying and treating these disorders by incorporating their assessment into routine well-woman care has the potential to positively affect the lives of a substantial number of women.

Our genetic makeup and environment interact. Evidence has emerged demonstrating preconception and prenatal exposure to toxic agents have a profound effect on reproductive health. We cannot change our genetics, but we can change our environment. Health providers can protect pregnancies from harmful exposures. Pregnancy is the most critical timewindow for human development, when any toxic exposure can cause lasting damage to brain development. Reproductive care professionals can provide useful information to patients and refer patients to appropriate specialists when hazardous exposure is identified. Clinical experience and expertise in communicating risks of treatment are transferable to environmental health.

Integrated care with mental health clinicians embedded in medical departments remains rare despite evidence of the need and effectiveness of such a model. Comprehensive, efficacious, and meaningful health care requires adequate attention be paid to the physiologic and the psychological symptoms of the patient. In the obstetrics/gynecology setting, myriad psychosocial concerns routinely present and cannot be adequately addressed in the current systems of care. The need is there, providers and patients have shown preference for such a structure, and the outcomes are promising. This article outlines common patient concerns in such settings and discusses possible interventions.

Advancements in cancer screening techniques have allowed for earlier detection of cancer at premalignant or early stages of disease. Several organizations have guidelines for screening strategies for breast, cervical, colon, and lung cancer. Ovarian cancer remains the deadliest cancer of the female reproductive tract; however, guidelines have yet to be shown effective in identifying ovarian cancer at earlier stages. It is important that providers familiarize themselves with up-to-date screening strategies in women at average risk and at increased risk of disease. The provider's role in guiding patients toward screening programs and counseling regarding risk reduction is one of the most important.

Section 2 - Maturity

Section 3 - Post Maturity

Carolyn J. Crandall

Osteoporosis is a common condition among postmenopausal women. Women 65 years and older should receive bone mineral testing; younger women should undergo risk assessment using a formal risk assessment tool to determine if they should receive bone density testing. Many pharmacologic agents are available to treat women with osteoporosis on bone density testing. Women with previous hip or vertebral fractures should also receive osteoporosis pharmacotherapy.

Section 4 - Conclusion

Mark S. DeFrancesco

The past 40 years have witnessed a major redesign of health care, largely driven by rampantly increasing costs and the perception of lack of better outcomes to justify those costs. Many demographic changes have also challenged the women's health care provider workforce, and evolving new payment systems are likewise a source of angst for these providers. Managed care is seeking to cut costs, and the challenge is to do so without sacrificing quality. Burnout is a new challenge in the present environment. There is now an opportunity to meet these challenges and provide the excellent care our patients deserve.

OBSTETRICS AND GYNECOLOGY CLINICS

Foreword

Optimal Women's Health Begins with Preventive Care

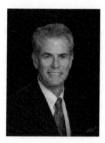

William F. Rayburn, MD, MBA, FACOG
Consulting Editor

Quality health care for women includes 2 fundamental elements: treatment for current illness and preventive care to lessen future health decline. I am pleased to present our first issue pertaining to preventive care in the *Obstetrics and Gynecology Clinics of North America.* The issue is well edited by the combined efforts of Dr Jeanne Conry and Dr Maureen Phipps, both leaders at the American College of Obstetricians and Gynecologists (ACOG). The many qualified authors present principles that support the development of recommendations for preventive care for women during their reproductive, mature, and postmature years.

This issue identifies preventions as being primary to keep disease from occurring (eg, immunization from communicable disease), secondary to detecting early asymptomatic disease (eg, screening), behavioral or lifestyle change counseling, chemoprevention, and as part of care for patients with preexisting disease. We are well aware of immunizations, especially for human papillomavirus vaccinations of adolescent girls for cervical cancer prevention. Screening tests in women often begin prenatally (such as for Down syndrome in fetuses and for maternal diabetes) and continue throughout life. Clinicians can give effective behavioral counseling at any time to motivate lifestyle changes, such as stopping smoking, eating a prudent diet, drinking alcohol in moderation, exercising regularly, and engaging in safe sexual practices. Chemoprevention is the use of drugs to prevent disease. A few examples would include long-acting contraception, preconception folate to reduce recurrent neural tube defects, and low-dose aspirin prophylaxis to reduce recurrent preeclampsia.

Screening is the early identification of potentially harmful conditions or risk factors. Three criteria are important when deciding what conditions justify screening: the burden of suffering caused by the condition; the effectiveness, safety, and cost of the preventive intervention; and the performance of the screening test. Preventive services are more likely to be discussed when a patient has an established relationship

Obstet Gynecol Clin N Am 46 (2019) xiii–xv
https://doi.org/10.1016/j.ogc.2019.05.002
0889-8545/19/© 2019 Published by Elsevier Inc.

obgyn.theclinics.com

with her obstetrician-gynecologist or other identified clinician. Creative solutions for delivering preventive care include either using patient databases with patient notification or incorporating care during patient visits for routine checkups, acute illness, or chronic conditions.

Specific recommendations for preventive women's health care are found throughout this issue. Current guidelines are provided about cardiovascular health and risk assessment (eg, hypertension, hyperlipidemia, obesity, diabetes, aspirin for prevention) and risk factors for the following cancers: breast, cervical, ovarian, and colorectal. Optimizing lifestyle is important to us all as we age. Several modalities to evaluate bone density are described for postmenopausal women with risk factors or those who are 65 or older. Accompanying psychosocial health concerns that deserve attention in this issue include depression, substance-related problems, and intimate partner violence. A unique article introduces the important backdrop of environmental exposures. The authors explain why exposures in the food we eat, air we breathe, water we drink, and products we use can impact the health of this and future generations.

Topics chosen in this issue were selected by important work generated from the *Women's Preventive Services Initiative (WPSI)*, a collaborative effort between health professional societies and consumer organizations focusing on women's health. This initiative requires a 5-year effort to develop, review, update, and disseminate recommendations for women's preventive health care services needed throughout their lifetime. In addition to the WPSI, I turn to the *US Preventive Services Task Force* for systematically reviewed and published evidence-based recommendations about multiple clinical preventive services considered in this issue. The *Centers for Disease Control and Prevention* makes annual recommendations for immunizations (influenza, Td/Tdap, human papillomavirus, zoster, pneumococcal, meningococcal, and hepatitis B) and for prevention and screening of sexually transmitted infections.

As women's health care providers, we should reach out to colleagues in other specialties, especially to underscore the importance of preconception care and reduce unplanned pregnancies. Prenatal and postpartum care involve a substantial amount of patient education and health promotion materials. This issue discusses routine patient education about optimizing health (diet, exercise and physical activity, oral health, avoidance of substances, immunizations, and preventive measures for other infections). When a medication needs to be taken, especially in the first trimester of pregnancy, the risks and benefits of taking versus not taking the drug require referencing the best available evidence from several resources.

The idea that screening programs can lead to harm is often foreign to our patients. Women's health care providers are encouraged to make sure that patients are aware of potential harms before any screening and consider any comorbidities when discussing screening. Potential harms associated with screening include anxiety produced with a positive diagnostic result (whether true or false), overdiagnosis of conditions that may be treated but not have become clinically apparent, and cost. As a suggestion, the provider may refocus the patient away from more intensive or time-consuming screening and toward other prevention activities that bring a higher likelihood of benefit. It is essential that clinicians present the benefits and harms in an understandable way, using absolute rather than relative risks and the strength of evidence.

As with all health care decisions, patient preferences are of prime importance. Printed or online patient education materials written in plain language at the 5th or 6th grade reading level (basics) or at the 10th to 12th grade level (beyond the basics) are available (eg, ACOG, UpToDate). Changes in national recommendations that decrease the frequency or intensity of screening and stopping screening for patients because of negligible or no additional benefit can lead to problematic discussions with patients. There are no strict guidelines for the optimal frequency of periodic visits, and minimal or no evidence on which to base the optimal frequency of specific recommendations. Last, the final article dealing with challenges in the era of coding and corporatization nicely summarizes the difficulties with compensation for preventive care.

In conclusion, optimal and continuing quality care begins with prevention. Dr Conry and Dr Phipps are to be commended for engaging experts who present important topics in women's preventive health. Their collective and collaborative wisdom reflects evidence from several professional associations. This timely issue will serve as a valuable resource for not only all obstetrician-gynecologists but also a diverse set of providers in women's health, including family physicians and internists, physician assistants, nurse practitioners, certified nurse-midwives, and public health nurses.

William F. Rayburn, MD, MBA, FACOG
University of New Mexico
School of Medicine
MSC 10 5580
1 University of New Mexico
Albuquerque, NM 87131-0001, USA

E-mail address:
wrayburn@salud.unm.edu

Preface

Every Woman, Every Time, Every Where

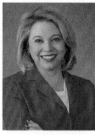
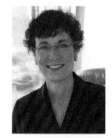

Jeanne A. Conry, MD, PhD   Maureen G. Phipps, MD, MPH
Editors

Investing in women's health leads to healthier women, families, communities, and populations, and this investment benefits the health of this and future generations. A commitment to women's health includes access to quality, affordable health care for women, preventive health care, continuity of care, and a focus on improving maternal and child health outcomes. Consistent with the World Health Organization's definition of health,[1] women's health is a state of complete physical, mental, and social well-being and not merely the absence of disease or infirmity. Unfortunately, whether we address global or national efforts, achieving women's health has fallen short of its potential. Embracing preventive care, including reproductive life planning, optimization of nutrition and exercise, screening for, prevention, and management of chronic diseases, immunizations, management of infectious diseases, and attention to psychological and behavioral health, has the potential to substantively improve women's overall health and well-being. In this issue of the *Obstetrics and Gynecology Clinics of North America*, we have engaged experts to present important topics in women's preventive health for the practicing clinician. The topics for this issue were informed by important work being generated from the Women's Preventive Services Initiative (WPSI).

The WPSI is a collaborative effort between health professional societies and consumer organizations that are focused on women's health. The goal of WPSI is to improve the health of all women throughout their life and to make recommendations that are applicable and accessible to all providers and health plans.[2] Women

Obstet Gynecol Clin N Am 46 (2019) xvii–xix
https://doi.org/10.1016/j.ogc.2019.05.001
0889-8545/19/© 2019 Published by Elsevier Inc.

obgyn.theclinics.com

should receive the highest quality care to the full extent intended in the Patient Protection and Affordable Care Act (ACA).[3] This focus on well-woman health care is particularly important given the ACA's strong provisions on women's health, including access to reproductive health planning and contraception, prenatal care, and preventive services, which include cancer and mental health screening. In addition, optimizing pregnancy and prenatal outcomes is dependent on preconception health and well-woman health, including "one key question": are you interested in conceiving this year?...For every woman, every time![4]

WPSI is a 5-year effort to develop, review, update, and disseminate recommendations for women's preventive health care services and identify needs throughout a woman's lifetime, from adolescence through adulthood into later maturity.[5] In order to ensure that women of all ages receive appropriate preventive health screenings, both health care providers and patients need reliable access to established recommendations. Dependable, consistent recommendations help clinicians determine which screenings and preventive health services they should routinely offer to patients.

In March 2016, Health Resources and Services Administration (HRSA) awarded a 5-year cooperative agreement to The American College of Obstetricians and Gynecologists (ACOG) to update the Institute of Medicine's 2011 *Clinical Preventive Services for Women: Closing the Gaps*[6] and subsequently to develop additional recommendations to enhance women's preventive services to improve overall health. The WPSI recognizes that women may seek guidance for preventive services from a diverse set of experts in women's health, including family physicians and internists, obstetrician-gynecologists, physician assistants, nurse practitioners, certified nurse-midwives, and public health nurses. WPSI's broad membership of specialty societies providing women's health care is poised to develop and share guidelines and to hold all entities accountable for optimizing the health and well-being of women. Efficient, effective guidelines established with evidence-based processes and vetted by women's health experts are necessary to optimize health care delivery and outcomes.

This issue of the *Obstetrics and Gynecology Clinics of North America* addresses the broader preventive health care needs of women. Topics range from cancer screening and reproductive health, to cardiovascular, bone, and urologic health. This is also a unique opportunity to introduce practicing women's health care clinicians to the important backdrop of environmental exposures. In this issue, the authors explain why exposures in the food we eat, the air we breathe, the water we drink, and the products we use can impact the health of this and future generations. A framework of environmental concerns can very well shape the health care of our generation.

As women's health care providers, we should make a point to reach out to colleagues in other specialties, to underscore the importance of preconception care, to reduce unplanned pregnancies, and to encourage everyone to consider the reproductive health of their female patients. Likewise, women's health care providers must understand that screening for broad health care needs, including cardiovascular, bone, metabolic, and urologic health as well as environmental exposures, are critical to our patients' overall health care needs and satisfaction.

Our collective and collaborative voice will be powerful, reflecting the combined wisdom of professional associations and women's health advocates to ultimately address the needs of women throughout the United States.

Jeanne A. Conry, MD, PhD
The Environmental Health Leadership Foundation
8204 Cantershire Way
Granite Bay, CA 95746, USA

Maureen G. Phipps, MD, MPH
Department of Obstetrics and Gynecology
Warren Alpert Medical School
of Brown University
Brown University School of Public Health
Women and Infants Hospital and Care
New England Health System
121 South Main Street
Providence, RI 02903, USA

E-mail addresses:
jeanneconry@gmail.com (J.A. Conry)
Maureen_Phipps@brown.edu (M.G. Phipps)

REFERENCES

1. World Health Organization. Basic documents. 45th edition, Supplement; 2006. Available at: https://www.who.int/governance/eb/who_constitution_en.pdf.
2. Available at: https://www.womenspreventivehealth.org/.
3. Available at: https://www.healthcare.gov/preventive-care-women/.
4. Conry J. Every woman, every time. Obstet Gynecol 2013;122(1):3–6.
5. Phipps MG, Son S, Zahn C, et al. Women's preventive services initiative's well-woman chart: a summary of preventive health recommendations for women. Obstet Gynecol 2019. [Epub ahead of print].
6. Institute of Medicine. Clinical preventive services for women: closing the gaps. Washington, DC: The National Academies Press; 2011. p. 236.

Section 1: Reproductive Age

Preconception Health
Changing the Paradigm on Well-woman Health

Diana E. Ramos, MD, MPH*

KEYWORDS

- Preconception health • Well-woman health • Unintended pregnancy • WPSI

KEY POINTS

- Preconception health is a continuum of well-woman health.
- Preconception health improves perinatal outcomes and community health.
- A public health approach is a good framework to promote preconception health and well-woman health.

BACKGROUND

Although advances in medicine and health care have made improvements in health outcomes, there is much more work to be done to address the health needs of the most vulnerable in the population, pregnant women and children. Increasing rates of maternal mortality, poor birth outcomes, and infant mortality embody the call to action for improvement. An investment in assuring the health of women, before pregnancy (preconception), will lead to improved health for women, children, and their families (**Fig. 1**). A paradigm shift of how health is thought of must occur to truly improve women's health and perinatal outcomes, moving beyond reactive care (seeking care when sick) and to preventive and preconception care.

Preconception health is centered on the assumption that a woman is planning to become pregnant. Many women do not plan for pregnancy, however, and may have medical conditions that have the potential to have a negative impact on pregnancy outcomes. Efforts have been aimed at curbing the high unintended pregnancy rate in the United States, currently 48%. The highest rates of unintended pregnancy are among low-income women, women aged 18 to 24, and women of color.[1] Unplanned pregnancies and late or no prenatal care are risk factors for poor pregnancy outcomes, including low birthweight, preterm births, and infant mortality. Early prenatal care has been recommended to improve perinatal outcomes.[2] In the United States,

Disclosure Statement: Nothing to disclose.
Department of Obstetrics and Gynecology, Keck School of Medicine, University of Southern California, Los Angeles, CA, USA
* PO Box 337, Laguna Beach, CA 92651.
E-mail address: drdramos@hotmail.com
; DrDianaRamosMD (D.E.R.)

Obstet Gynecol Clin N Am 46 (2019) 399–408
https://doi.org/10.1016/j.ogc.2019.04.001
obgyn.theclinics.com

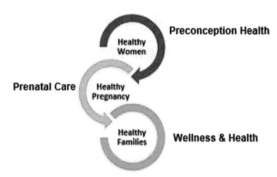

Fig. 1. Healthy women all the time: preconception health's impact on improving healthy families.

77% of women initiate prenatal care in the first trimester; this is close to the Healthy People 2020 goal of 77.9%.[3] But, disparities in obtaining early prenatal care exist among less educated, younger women and in black, non-Hispanic, and Native Hawaiian and other Pacific Islander women.[4]

When comparing the US unintended pregnancy rates with those worldwide, they are consistent with the global rate of 41%.[5] The United States ranks lower, however, than most Western countries when analyzing maternal and infant outcomes. The Mother's Index (MI), which assesses the well-being of mothers and children in 179 countries, is one measure for global comparison. The Norway, Finland, and Iceland MIs ranked as the top 3 whereas the United States ranked thirty-third.[6] One common denominator among countries ranking above the US is the provision of universal health care, which provides wellness and preventive medical services. Therefore, women with unintended pregnancies in countries with a high MI have had access to lifelong health care, including during the preconception period.

NEW PARADIGM FOR PRECONCEPTION HEALTH AND WELL-WOMAN HEALTH

A new paradigm focusing on lifelong continuum of health—healthy women all the time—which, when a woman is planning her reproductive life, is called preconception and interconception health (**Fig. 2**), is now more achievable through implementation of the

The Affordable Care Act (ACA)—the health insurance reform legislation passed by Congress and signed into law in 2010—requires health plans to cover preventive services and zero out-of-pocket costs. Women-specific covered benefits are listed in **Box 1**, many of which can be considered preconception care for women who become pregnant.[7]

A public awareness survey of ACA health benefits demonstrated 38.6% of women were aware of the covered benefits but often were not aware of what they should have done.[8] The Women's Preventive Services Initiative (WPSI), a federally supported collaborative program led by the American College of Obstetricians and Gynecologists, continues to review and recommend updates to the Women's Preventive Services Guidelines, also a part of the covered benefits for women.

WELL-WOMAN HEALTH

A well-woman visit focuses on promoting and maintaining health over the course of a woman's lifetime through preventive health care.[9–12] Caveats to the well-woman visit

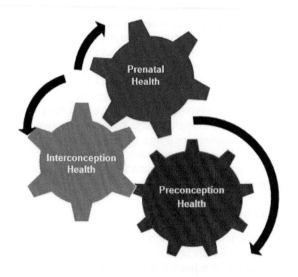

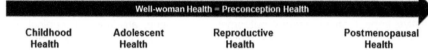

Fig. 2. Preconception health and interconception health are part of the well-woman health continuum.

include that a visit can be spread out over several visits and delivered by members of a health care team, not just the physician. During the well-woman visit, the opportunity exists to assess her reproductive life plan. As Nichole Tyson's article, "Reproductive Health: Options, Strategies, and Empowerment of Women," in this issue, discusses,

---

Box 1
Women's preventive services recommended by the Institute of Medicine to be covered under the Affordable Care Act

Well-woman visits

Screening for gestational diabetes

Human papillomavirus testing

Counseling and screening for sexually transmitted infections

Counseling and screening for HIV

Contraceptive methods and counseling[a]

Breastfeeding support, supplies, and counseling

Screening and counseling for interpersonal and domestic violence

  [a] See *Federal Register Notice: Religious Exemptions and Accommodations for Coverage of Certain Preventive Services Under the Affordable Care Act.*
  Adapted from Health Resources & Services Administration (HRSA). Women's preventive services guidelines. Available at: https://www.hrsa.gov/womens-guidelines/index.html. Accessed April 4, 2019.

advantages of assessing reproductive intention at every medical encounter. Health care providers should discuss reproductive plans, prescribe contraception if appropriate, and address chronic conditions that could compromise maternal health. Women should contact their provider if they have any concerns during their pregnancy. If a pregnancy is desired, the visit becomes a preconception health visit (**Fig. 3**). Preconception recommendations are based on her medical conditions.

Recommendations for Well-Woman Care—A Well-Woman Chart is a resource developed by the WPSI that summarizes age-based preventive service recommendations for women from adolescence into maturity. The women's preventive service chart summarizes the evidence-based assessments, screening, evaluation and counseling, and immunizations based on age and risk factors (www.womenspreventivehealth.org/wellwomanchart).

PRECONCEPTION HEALTH

The components of preconception health have been suggested by various organizations but preconception health care is different for every person because of personal health needs. Based on a person's individual health, the health care provider suggests a course of treatment or follow-up care as needed. The common denominator lies in addressing any health behaviors or health conditions that can have a negative impact on pregnancy outcomes; in essence, any and all medical and behavioral conditions can be included. Following is a review of general suggested components derived from the Centers for Disease Control and Prevention (CDC) and the Office on Women's Health. Depending on the positive screens identified by the provider, resources can be provided to address the issues for which she screens positive (**Box 2**).

FOLIC ACID

The recommended 400 μg of folic acid every day, starting at least 1 month prior to conception, can reduce the risk for neural tube defects, spina bifida, or anencephaly by 50% to 70%[13,14] Folic acid is a water-soluble vitamin, and any excess consumed is rapidly excreted in the urine. Folic acid is important in cells that are undergoing high replication, such as in hair, nails, skin, and an embryo. Sources of folate include a supplement and foods. Foods with high folate content include green leafy vegetables,

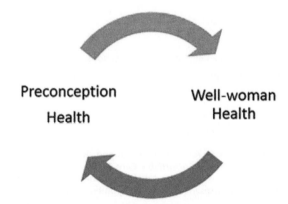

Preconception Health   **Well-woman Health**

Fig. 3. The relationship between preconception health and well-woman health.

| Box 2 |
| Preconception health elements |

Take folic acid every day

Stop drinking alcohol, smoking, and using street drugs

Assure good control of medical condition

Have vaccinations up to date

Avoid toxic substances or materials that could cause infection

Maintain a healthy weight

Encourage mental health

Promote violence prevention

Data from U.S. Department of Health & Human Services. Office on Women's Health (OWH). Preconception health. Available at: https://www.womenshealth.gov/pregnancy/you-get-pregnant/preconception-health. Accessed December 29, 2018; and Centers for Disease Control and Prevention (CDC). Before pregnancy. Planning for pregnancy. Available at: https://www.cdc.gov/preconception/planning.html. Accessed January 17, 2019.

legumes, and foods fortified with folate—breads, breakfast cereals, and corn masa flour. Obtaining folate through a daily supplement and eating fortified foods is an easy way to obtain the daily recommended amount. In the United States, Hispanic women have the highest rate of neural tube defects; they are least likely to consume foods fortified with folic acid or to know that taking a vitamin with folic acid can decrease the risk for neural tube defects. For women who have had a pregnancy affected with a neural tube defect or on certain seizure medications, the recommended amount of folic acid is 4 mg daily at least 1 month before pregnancy.[15]

ALCOHOL, SMOKING, AND STREET DRUGS

There is no safe amount of alcohol to drink during pregnancy, especially because many women may not know they are pregnant. A consequence of alcohol consumption during pregnancy is fetal alcohol syndrome, which can cause growth problems, intellectual disability, behavioral problems, and abnormal facial features.[16]

In 2013, approximately 1 in 5 women smoked in the 3 months before pregnancy, and approximately 1 in 10 smoked during the last 3 months of pregnancy.[17] Nicotine is only 1 of 4000 toxic chemicals that can pass from a pregnant woman to her fetus. Nicotine causes blood vessels to narrow, so less oxygen and fewer nutrients reach the fetus. Nicotine also damages a fetus' brain and lungs. E-cigarettes contain harmful nicotine plus flavoring and a propellant that may not be safe for a fetus. E-cigarettes are not safe substitutes for cigarettes and should not be used during pregnancy.

Use of street drugs, including heroin, cocaine, methamphetamines, opioids, and prescription drugs taken for a nonmedical reason, is a widespread problem in the United States. Approximately 1 in 20 women uses illegal drugs during pregnancy. Birth defects, low birth, prematurity, fetal death, and miscarriages are associated with the use of street drugs. Although it is legal in some states, marijuana should not be used in any form during pregnancy. Marijuana used during pregnancy is associated with attention and behavioral problems in children. Marijuana may increase the risk of stillbirth, low weight, and delayed infant developmental milestones. Misusing opioids during pregnancy is associated with placental abruption, fetal growth problems, preterm birth, and stillbirth.[17]

MEDICAL CONDITIONS

Chronic conditions, such as high blood pressure, diabetes, heart disease, Thyroid disorder, seizure disorder asthma, and obesity may put women at higher risk of pregnancy complications. Approximately half of Americans are living with at least 1 chronic disease.[18] Chronic medical conditions are more common or severe for minority groups (specifically, non-Hispanic blacks, Hispanics, American Indians, Alaska Natives, Asians, Native Hawaiians, and Pacific Islanders).[19] The most common cause of maternal death in the country now is complications occurring as a result of a mother's preexisting, chronic condition (such conditions are attributed to half of all maternal deaths in the United States).[20]

Women with underlying medical conditions should be sure that they are under control and being treated. These may include sexually transmitted infections, diabetes, thyroid disease, phenylketonuria, seizure disorders, high blood pressure, arthritis, eating disorders, and chronic diseases.[21]

MEDICATIONS

Certain medicines, such as prescription medications, vitamin supplements, herbal remedies, and over-the-counter medications, can be teratogenic. Review of medications is important to know if a medication should be stopped or if an alternative, non-teratogenic medication can be substituted.[21]

VACCINATIONS

Some vaccinations are recommended before pregnancy, such as the rubella vaccine. Knowing which vaccines are needed before pregnancy can provide immunity during pregnancy and prevent fetal infection and consequences.[16] The WPSI follows the CDC vaccination recommendations.

AVOID TOXIC SUBSTANCES OR MATERIALS THAT CAN CAUSE INFECTION

Toxic substances, such as lead or mercury and other environmental contaminants at work or at home, such as synthetic chemicals, metals, fertilizer, pesticides, and cat or rodent feces, should be avoided. DeNicola and McCue give a thorough overview of the impact of environmental toxics on health that can lead to adverse outcomes in pregnancy and in maternal or child health, in Kristen A. Matteson's and Kate Zaluski's article, "Menstrual Health as a Part of Preventive Health Care," in this issue. These substances can hurt the reproductive systems of men and women. Some may lead to infertility and others can cause disease leading to miscarriages or birth defects.[16,22]

HEALTHY WEIGHT

As Elizabeth A. Hoover and Judette M. Louis' article, "Optimizing Health: Weight, Exercise, and Nutrition in Pregnancy and Beyond," in this issue discusses, being overweight or obese contributes to pregnancy and childbirth complications, including high blood pressure, preeclampsia, preterm birth, and gestational diabetes. There also is a higher risk of birth defects, especially neural tube defects.[16]

Lifelong complications include an increased risk of heart disease, type 2 diabetes mellitus, and certain cancers (endometrial, breast, and colon).[23,24] Overall, African Americans and Hispanics have the highest rate of obesity in the United States.

MENTAL HEALTH

In the United States, approximately 1 in 2 people have a mental health diagnosis in their lifetime.[25] Mental illnesses, such as depression, are the third most common cause of hospitalization in the United States for those 18 to 44 years old.[26,27] Adults living with serious mental illness die on average 25 years earlier than others. In a pregnant woman, mental health conditions during and after pregnancy have an impact not only on the health of the mother but on the birth outcomes and child behavior. There is a higher rate of mental health disorders, such as depression, which can affect the health and well-being of women and their families. It is estimated that 20% of women suffer from mood or anxiety disorders. Approximately 1 in 9 pregnant women had symptoms of major depression in 2013, only half of these women received treatment.[28,29]

For patients needing to be on medication, reviewing the risk/benefit of medications should be part of the mental health assessment. Priya Batra's article, "Integrated Mind/Body Care in Women's Health: A Focus On Well-Being, Mental Health and Relationships," in this issue, points out the successful team-based care that can treat depression and anxiety.

VIOLENCE PREVENTION

Approximately 1 in 4 adult women (23%) experience severe physical violence (ie, being kicked, beaten, chocked, or burned on purpose or having a weapon used against her) from an intimate partner in their lifetime. Intimate partner violence is especially prevalent among women of reproductive age and can contribute, among many other conditions, to pregnancy complications, unintended pregnancy, and sexually transmitted infections.[30] Screening all women and offering support along with referral options should be provided. Intimate partner violence is more common than diabetes in pregnancy but is not screened at the same level.[31]

OPERATIONALIZING PRECONCEPTION HEALTH

The groundwork for the content and coverage of well-woman health, which becomes preconception health when a woman plans on becoming pregnant, has been established through the ACA initial Institute of Medicine women's health recommendations and continues through the WPSI well-woman health recommendations. What is needed to operationalize and increase consumer and provider awareness of preconception health is a framework for promotion and provision. Health providers can recognize that preconception health is simply well-woman's health and women know the importance of striving for good health at all the time and if they are planning on becoming pregnant.

A public health framework operationalizes the continuum of well-woman health and preconception health, and it is a framework familiar to health care providers and consumers. Primary prevention focuses on decreasing disease before it occurs, through immunizations, education on healthy habits, and legislation to ban or control the use of hazardous products (eg, asbestos) or to mandate safe and healthy practices (eg, use of seatbelts and bike helmets). Secondary prevention focuses on screening, detecting and treating early disease before the onset of signs and symptoms, for example, blood pressure check. Tertiary prevention efforts focus on preventing progression of disease once diagnosed, that is, rehabilitation.[32]

The aim of preconception health is primary prevention, when possible. Recommendations, such as daily intake of folic acid, emphasize the opportunity to prevent neural tube defects in women who are deficient. Encouraging vaccinations, not smoking, and avoiding the use of alcohol or street drugs also are primary preventions. When providing education and prevention messaging, attention should be paid not only to literacy level, language, and culture but also the method in which content is delivered. Reproductive-age women obtain health messaging through social media, videos, and other interactive platforms. Targeting and tailoring information on preconception messaging with these platforms can have a higher probability of reach. Text messaging can provide preventive information and reinforce preconception, while wellness messaging improves health behaviors.[33]

Secondary prevention components of women's wellness health include screening for sexually transmitted infections, human immunodeficiency virus (HIV), human papillomavirus, and domestic violence. These secondary prevention issues, when addressed around the preconception period, have the potential to prevent neonatal comorbidities, such as congenital syphilis, chlamydia, and HIV, and the negative impacts on an infant born into a home where domestic violence is present. Any of these components screened preconceptionally has as a consequence of prevention of at-risk infants being born preterm and/or of low birth weight. Once the presence of disease has been diagnosed, the author moves on to tertiary care, where the focus is preventing disease progression. Chronic hypertension illustrates how encouraging good control and managing with needed medication help prevent disease progression and comorbidities, such as heart disease.[34]

SUMMARY

Focusing on well-woman's health, and referring to it as preconception health when a woman is planning a pregnancy, has the potential to improve the health of women, infants, and families. Evidence has demonstrated improved outcomes for infants (lower rates of preterm births and infant mortality) and mothers (lower maternal morbidity and mortality). With approximately half of all births in the United States unplanned, changing the focus from just preconception health to a continuum of lifelong well-woman care is needed. Having a goal of healthy women at all times so that in the event a woman becomes pregnant, optimal health and well-being are present from the start. Focusing on healthy women all the time has the potential to eliminate some racially and socioeconomically based negative perinatal outcomes. A public health approach provides a familiar framework for implementation and partnership between providers, consumers, and public health partners. Together health will be reframed to focus on prevention and lifelong health. Over time, perinatal, maternal, and family health will improve and the intergenerational health in the United States will be on par with that in other countries.

REFERENCES

1. Finer LB, Zolna MR. Declines in unintended pregnancy in the United States, 2008–2011. N Engl J Med 2016;374(9):843–52.
2. Prenatal care. Available at: https://www.nichd.nih.gov/health/topics/pregnancy/conditioninfo/prenatal-care. Accessed December 22, 2018.
3. Healthy People 2020 [Internet]. Washington, DC: US Department of Health and Human Services, Office of Disease Prevention and Health Promotion. Available at: https://www.healthypeople.gov/2020/topics-objectives/topic/maternal-infant-and-child-health/objectives. Accessed January 5, 2019.

4. Osterman MJK, Martin JA. Timing and adequacy of prenatal care in the United States, 2016. National vital Statistics Reports, vol. 67. Hyattsville (MD): National Center for Health Statistics; 2018. no 3.
5. Singh S, Sedgh G, Hussain R, et al. Unintended pregnancy: worldwide levels, trends, and outcomes. Stud Fam Plann 2010;41(4):241–50.
6. The Urban Disadvantage State of the World's Mothers 2015. Available at: https://www.savethechildren.org/content/dam/usa/reports/advocacy/sowm/sowm-2015.pdf. Accessed January 4, 2019.
7. Women's preventive services recommended by IOM to be covered under affordable care act. Available at: https://www.hrsa.gov/womens-guidelines/index.html. Accessed April 4, 2019.
8. Williams JAR, Ortiz SE. Examining public knowledge and preferences for adult preventive services coverage. PLoS One 2017;12(12):e0189661.
9. Conry B. Well-woman task force: components of the well-woman visit. Obstet Gynecol 2015;126:697–701. Available at: https://journals.lww.com/greenjournal/Fulltext/2015/10000/Well_Woman_Task_Force__Components_of_the.2.aspx.
10. WPSI. Available at: https://www.womenspreventivehealth.org/wellwomanchart/. Accessed January 17, 2019.
11. Pre-conception Healh. Available at: https://www.womenshealth.gov/pregnancy/you-get-pregnant/preconception-health. Accessed December 29, 2018.
12. Preconception health. Available at: https://www.cdc.gov/preconception/planning.html. Accessed January 17, 2019.
13. Czeizel AE, Dudas I. Prevention of the first occurrence of neural-tube defects by periconceptional vitamin supplementation. N Engl J Med 1992;327:1832–5.
14. Laurence KM, James N, Miller MH, et al. Double-blind randomized controlled trial of folate treatment before conception to prevent recurrence of neural-tube defects. BMJ 1981;282:1509–11.
15. Folic Acid: CDC. Available at: https://www.cdc.gov/ncbddd/folicacid/recommendations.html. Accessed January 18, 2019.
16. Planning for pregnancy. Available at: https://www.cdc.gov/preconception/planning.html#ref. Accessed January 17, 2019.
17. ACOG FAQ tobacco, alcohol, drugs, and pregnancy. Available at: https://www.acog.org/Patients/FAQs/Tobacco-Alcohol-Drugs-and-Pregnancy. Accessed January 24, 2019.
18. Center for Disease Control. Chronic disease overview. Available at: http://www.cdc.gov/nccdphp/overview.htm. Accessed January 25, 2019.
19. Finding solutions to health disparities at a glance. Available at: https://www.cdc.gov/chronicdisease/resources/publications/aag/reach.htm. Accessed April 4, 2019.
20. Admon LK, Winkelman TNA, Moniz MH. Disparities in chronic conditions among women hospitalized for delivery in the United States, 2005–2014. Obstet Gynecol 2017;130(6):1319–26. The Green Journal.
21. Good Health Before Pregnancy. Prepregnancy care FAQ056 2018. Available at: https://www.acog.org/Patients/FAQs/Good-Health-Before-Pregnancy-Prepregnancy-Care#affect. Accessed April 4, 2019.
22. Good Health Before Pregnancy. Pre-pregnancy care FAQ056. 2018. Available at: https://www.acog.org/Patients/FAQs/Good-Health-Before-Pregnancy-Prepregnancy-Care#affect. Accessed December 20, 2018.
23. Moos MK, Dunlop AL, Jack BW, et al. Healthier women, healthier reproductive outcomes: recommendations for the routine care of all women of reproductive age. Am J Obstet Gynecol 2008;199(6, Supplement B):S280–9.

24. Prevalence of self –reported obesity among U.S. Adults by race/ethnicity, state and territory, BRFSS, 2015 2017. Available at: https://www.cdc.gov/obesity/data/prevalence-maps.html. Accessed April 4, 2019.

25. CDC Mental Health. Available at: https://www.cdc.gov/mentalhealth/data_publications/index.htm. Accessed April 4, 2019.

26. Parks J, Svendsen D, Singer P, et al. Morbidity and mortality in people with serious mental.pdf. External. Alexandria (VA): National Association of State Mental Health Program Directors Medical Directors Council; 2006.

27. Kessler RC, Angermeyer M, Anthony JC, et al. Lifetime prevalence and age-of-onset distributions of mental disorders in the World Health Organization'o World Mental Health Survey Initiative. World Psychiatry 2007;6(3):168–76.

28. Flynn HA, Blow FC, Marcus SM. Rates and predictors of depression treatment among pregnant women in hospital-affiliated obstetrics practices. Gen Hosp Psychiatry 2006;28(No. 4):289–329.

29. At a glance 2016 maternal health advancing the health of mothers in the 21st century. Available at: https://www.cdc.gov/chronicdisease/resources/publications/aag/pdf/2016/aag-maternal-health.pdf. Accessed January 4, 2019.

30. ACOG Number 518, February 2012 Intimate Partner Violence. Available at: https://www.acog.org/Clinical-Guidance-and-Publications/Committee-Opinions/Committee-on-Health-Care-for-Underserved-Women/Intimate-Partner-Violence. Accessed December 20, 2018.

31. Alhusen JL, Ray E, Sharps P, et al. Intimate partner violence during pregnancy: maternal and neonatal outcomes. J Womens Health (Larchmt) 2015;24(1):100–6.

32. Picture of America. CDC. Available at: https://www.cdc.gov/pictureofamerica/pdfs/picture_of_america_prevention.pdfcan be understood and implemented. Accessed December 22, 2018.

33. FAMILIA : Los Angeles County Department of Public Health. Available at: https://admin.publichealth.lacounty.gov/mch/ReproductiveHealth/FAMILIA/FAMILIAhome.htm. Accessed January 2, 2019.

34. Picture of America CDC. Available at: https://www.cdc.gov/pictureofamerica/pdfs/picture_of_america_prevention.pdf. Accessed January 15, 2019.

Reproductive Health
Options, Strategies, and Empowerment of Women

Nichole A. Tyson, MD[a,b,*]

KEYWORDS

- Contraception • Birth control • LARC • IUD • Implant • Shot • Birth control pills
- Emergency contraception

KEY POINTS

- Ensuring access to a variety of contraceptives is essential to promote the health and autonomy of women.
- Contraception counseling should begin before a person becomes sexually active; occur at routine adolescent, well-woman, and prenatal visits; and continue to address goals and contraceptive needs as a person traverses through her reproductive career.
- The implant and intrauterine devices (IUDs) are top-tier contraceptives because of their efficacy, low side effect profile, and ease of use.
- The Centers for Disease Control and Prevention (CDC) Medical Eligibility Criteria (MEC) guideline and Selected Practice Recommendations (SPR) are superb resources that provide safety guidance and information on the contraception methods available in the United States.
- To minimize barriers and optimize pregnancy prevention, health care providers should prescribe and provide contraception and encourage initiation in a single visit.

INTRODUCTION

"When women are able to time and space their pregnancies, they are more likely to advance their education and earn an income–and they're more likely to have healthy children." Melinda Gates eloquently asserts that not only does contraception help people plan their families but ensuring access to contraception is essential to promote the health and autonomy of women.

Disclosure Statement: The author has nothing to disclose.
[a] Department of Obstetrics and Gynecology, The Permanente Medical Group, 1600 Eureka Road, Medical Office Building C, 3rd Floor, Roseville, CA 95661, USA; [b] UC Davis Medical Center, Sacramento, CA, USA
* Department of Obstetrics and Gynecology, The Permanente Medical Group, 1600 Eureka Road, Medical Office Building C, 3rd Floor, Roseville, CA 95661.
E-mail address: nichole.tyson@kp.org
; @NicholeATyson (N.A.T.)

Contraception helps women of all ages. Contraception permits young girls the opportunity to delay pregnancy and complete their physical and mental growth and development. This is particularly important for those girls who may be at increased risk of health problems and death from early childbearing. Contraception gives women the opportunity to complete their education and to pursue and fulfill their career goals. Contraception reduces teenage pregnancies, which are associated with more detrimental outcomes than pregnancies in older cohorts. Contraception allows people to control and make educated decisions about their sexual and reproductive health. Access to contraception reduces the need for abortion, improves the health of the teenager, and reduces significant risks associated with teenage births. Pregnant adolescents are more likely to have preterm or low-birth-weight babies, and babies born to adolescents have higher rates of neonatal mortality. Preventing teenage births has long-term implications for the individual patient, their families, and communities as a whole.

Access to birth control also helps adult women. Contraception reinforces autonomy to determine the number of pregnancies, if any, and spacing of children in one's family. Contraception helps women who may face health risks caused by pregnancy. It helps women limit their family size and minimize risk for themselves and their other children. Drs Rachel A. Newman and Afshan B. Hameed's article, "Matters of the Heart: Cardiovascular Health in Women Throughout their Lifetimes," in this issue, points out that evidence suggests that women who have more than four children are at increased risk of maternal mortality and long-term cardiovascular disease. Access to effective contraception helps women avoid closely spaced and poorly timed pregnancies and births. These unintended pregnancies contribute to high infant and maternal mortality rates. Additionally, infants of mothers who die in childbirth have a greater risk of poor health and early death themselves.

Contraception has a significant impact on many social and global factors. Contraceptive methods also serve to regulate menstrual disorders as described by Drs Kristen A. Matteson and Kate Zaluski's article, "Menstrual Health as a part of Preventive Health Care," in this issue. Having fewer children allows families to invest more in each child, and children who have fewer siblings often obtain higher educational achievements. Contraception is an essential component to reducing growth of the population, the negative sequalae impacting individuals and their communities, and promoting a sustainable environment and global health.

REPRODUCTIVE WINDOW AND UNPLANNED PREGNANCIES

The average woman in the United States uses contraception for 30 years to obtain her family goal of two children.[1] It is estimated that couples who do not use contraception have an 85% chance of getting pregnant in 1 year.[2] As Dr Diana E. Ramos's article, "Preconception Health: Changing the Paradigm on Well-Woman Health," in this issue points out, unfortunately, a gap in contraception access and use persists today, because latest estimates reveal that approximately half of the pregnancies in the United States are unintended.[3] When accounting for unintended pregnancies, those who do not use birth control consistently (20%) or at all (15%) account for 90% of unintended pregnancies in the United States. Most (70%) women who use contraception correctly and effectively account for only 5% of the unintended pregnancies.[4]

EFFICACY

The terminology of contraceptive efficacy is complex. Contraceptive failure rates are defined as the percentage of users who will become pregnant within the first

12 months of initiating use. Perfect-use failure rates apply to those who use a method consistently and correctly. Typical-use failure rates consider the inconsistent and incorrect use by contraceptive users. Contraceptive efficacy is routinely described in terms of a Pearl Index, which indicates the number of contraceptive failures per 100 woman-years of exposure. The contraceptive implant and the intrauterine devices (IUD) are the most effective reversible contraceptive methods available, with failure rates of around 1% for both perfect and typical use. These methods have low typical-use failure rates because they do not require user intervention. The implant and IUDs, or long-acting contraceptive methods (eg, long-acting reversible contraception [LARC]), are top-tier contraceptives and are colloquially referred to as the "get them and forget them" options because of their lack of need for regular compliance.[5]

When counseling patients, the relationship between typical and perfect use can help in contraceptive selection and optimizing best choice for each individual patient at her current time in life. Visual flow charts (**Fig. 1**) have been designed to optimize patient counseling reflecting efficacy of the methods.

Effectiveness is not the only factor women consider when making their contraceptive decision. Because of patient's individual beliefs, experiences, goals, motivations,

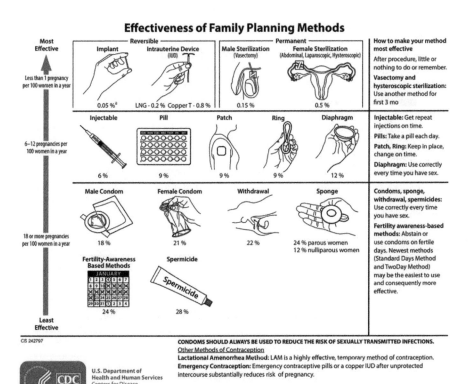

Fig. 1. Contraceptive efficacy. [a] The percentages indicate the number out of every 100 women who experienced an unintended pregnancy within the first year of typical use of each contraceptive method. (*From* Centers for Disease Control and Prevention (CDC). Reproductive health. Available at: https://www.cdc.gov/reproductivehealth/contraception/unintendedpregnancy/pdf/Contraceptive_methods_508.pdf.)

and knowledge, the contraceptive decision is a complex and unique one. Some studies have shown that when contraceptive counselors highlight the most effective methods, patients are more likely to use them.[6] However, although some patients may not be interested in becoming pregnant, they are simultaneously apprehensive about using birth control to prevent pregnancy. The reluctance to using birth control has been shown to be analogous to approaching patient education on other important health topics, such as smoking cessation and weight management.[7]

Contraception education and counseling by health care providers is a key component to every reproductive age women's health visit. Discussing all effective contraceptive options during these health care visits should ideally begin before a person becomes sexually active. Contraceptive counseling should occur at routine teenage, well-woman, and prenatal visits. The counseling should be fluid and flexible, continuing to address goals and contraceptive needs as a person traverses her reproductive career. Contraception counseling contributes to women becoming more likely to use contraception and ultimately has positive impacts on her health.[8]

SAFETY

In 1996 the World Health Organization, in collaboration with many international family planning agencies, published the first edition of the Medical Eligibility Criteria (MEC) for Contraceptive Use.[9] In 2010, the Centers for Disease Control and Prevention (CDC) adapted this guideline to address specific health care situations, medical conditions, and contraceptive options that pertain to patients in the United States. This MEC guideline and comprehensive table was updated in late 2015 and is considered the premier guide on the safety of contraceptive methods. The MEC outlines categories of risk for all available contraceptive methods in the United States (**Table 1**).

In 2013, to further optimize contraception use, the CDC Selected Practice Recommendations (SPR) provided additional guidance on the who, how, and when to use various contraception methods available in the United States.[10] The SPR provides guidance on whom should be screened for contraception, how and when to start a method, and how to manage common issues that arise. The SPR also provides specialized counsel on optimizing contraceptive use in special patient populations, such as adolescents.

Table 1	
Categories of medical eligibility criteria for contraceptive use	
Category	
1	A condition for which there is no restriction for the use of the contraceptive method.
2	A condition for which the advantages of using the method generally outweigh the theoretic or proven risk.
3	A condition for which the theoretic or proven risks usually outweigh the advantages of using the method. Use of this method is not usually recommended unless other or more appropriate methods are not available or acceptable.
4	A condition that represents an unacceptable health risk if the contraceptive method is used.

Adapted from Centers for Disease Control and Prevention (CDC). U.S. medical eligibility criteria for contraceptive use, 2016. MMWR Morb Mortal Wkly Rep 2016;65:1–104.

TIMING

Before starting a contraceptive method, the SPR has outlined an assessment for "ruling out" pregnancy without reliance on pregnancy tests (**Box 1**). Urine pregnancy tests are useful, but pregnancy tests are not always available and may be limited by the interval between fertilization and human chorionic gonadotropic detection in the urine. It takes at least 2 weeks following ovulation before a negative urine or blood pregnancy test can conclusively rule out pregnancy. Additionally, note that human chorionic gonadotropic is typically detectable in blood and urine for several weeks after a spontaneous or induced abortion and should not be considered indicative of an ongoing viable pregnancy. All methods other than IUD (if not using Paragard for emergency contraception [EC]) can be started immediately. Several concerns arise when considering initiating contraception. First, many women and providers are concerned about teratogenesis of birth control if they were to be pregnant when they start a method. It is reassuring to know that there is no evidence that hormonal contraception is harmful to a developing fetus.[11] Second, the "when to start a method" question is often perplexing for patients and providers. Quick start, immediate initiation of a method, was originally developed with combined hormonal oral contraceptive pills and showed to initially improve continuation rates of hormonal contraception.[12–14] The quick start method can safely be applied to the initiation of nearly any hormonal contraceptive method. If a patient does begin a contraceptive method when they are early in pregnancy, a delay in pregnancy diagnosis could delay a desired termination in pregnancy or timely prenatal care. Thus, if quick start methods are initiated, many clinicians order a urine pregnancy test 2 to 4 weeks later to screen for possible early pregnancy.

Unlike other contraceptive methods, IUDs, if inserted during pregnancy, can cause pregnancy complications. When considering timing of placing an IUD, reviewing criteria to reasonably rule out pregnancy (see **Box 1**) is advised. Should the person not meet the criteria for IUD placement, counseling and joint decision making should be obtained to consider the options: delaying placement, providing an interim method of birth control, or placing the IUD with the patient understanding the risks and benefits of insertion (**Box 2**).

Box 1
How to rule out pregnancy

A health care provider can be reasonably certain that a woman is not pregnant if she has no symptoms or signs of pregnancy and meets any *one* of the following criteria:
- Is ≤7 days after the start of normal menses
- Has not had sexual intercourse since the start of last normal menses
- Has been correctly and consistently using hormonal contraception or condoms
- Is ≤7 days after spontaneous or induced abortion
- Is within 4 weeks postpartum
- Is fully or nearly fully breastfeeding (exclusively breastfeeding or most [≥85%] feeds are breastfeeds), amenorrheic, and <6 months postpartum

If a provider cannot reasonably rule out pregnancy, *offer interim contraception.*

Although pregnancy tests are routinely performed before IUD insertion, a pregnancy test cannot detect a pregnancy resulting from recent intercourse. If pregnancy cannot be reasonably ruled out, the woman should be provided with another contraceptive method until the provider can reasonably be sure that she is not pregnant and can then insert the IUD.

Adapted from Centers for Disease Control and Prevention (CDC). U.S. selected practice recommendations for contraceptive use, 2016. MMWR Morb Mortal Wkly Rep 2016;65:1–66.

Box 2
Counseling regarding same-day IUD insertion in the setting of recent unprotected sex

I have counseled the patient that today's negative pregnancy test does not identify a pregnancy that started less than 2 weeks ago. Given that she has had unprotected sex in the last 2 weeks, there is a small chance of early unidentified pregnancy. I counseled her that she can choose to have the IUD inserted today because her overall chance for pregnancy is low or she can choose to return for an IUD insertion after 2 weeks of using condoms or another contraceptive method (pill, patch, shot, ring) as her birth control method. Inserting the IUD today, if she is early pregnant, could accidently cause a miscarriage or could increase her chance for preterm birth if she chose to keep the pregnancy. She is aware that she needs to repeat her pregnancy test in 2 to 3 weeks to confirm that she is not pregnant.

To minimize barriers and optimize pregnancy prevention, health care providers should prescribe and encourage contraceptive initiation in a single visit. Sexually transmitted infection testing can occur on the same day as contraceptive provision and LARC placement. Women do not require cervical cancer screening for contraceptive prescription or LARC placement.[10,15] Algorithms can guide providers on contraceptive candidacy and timing (**Figs. 2** and **3**).

CONTRACEPTIVE OPTIONS IN THE UNITED STATES

The Women's Preventive Services Initiative recommends that the full range of female-controlled US Food and Drug Administration–approved contraceptive methods, effective family planning practices, and sterilization procedures be available as part of contraceptive care.[16,17] The full range of contraceptive methods for women currently include: implantable rods (Nexplanon), progesterone-containing IUDs (all durations and doses) and copper T IUD (**Table 2**), the shot or injection (medroxyprogesterone acetate), the contraceptive patch, vaginal contraceptive ring, combined oral contraceptive pills (extended or continuous use), progestin-only contraceptive pills, female and male sterilization, female and male condoms, diaphragms, sponges, cervical caps, and spermicide. Additionally, instruction in fertility awareness-based methods, including the lactation amenorrhea method, although less effective, should be provided for women desiring alternative contraceptive methods (**Table 3**).

Emergency Contraception

EC is an important component of contraception counseling. EC involves using a nonabortifacient hormonal medication within 120 hours after unprotected or underprotected intercourse. Indications for EC include any situation in which sexual intercourse is unprotected, including reproductive coercion, sexual assault, or contraceptive method failure. Mechanisms are thought to inhibit or delay ovulation, interfere with tubal transport and fertilization, prevent implantation, or cause regression of the corpus luteum. The use of levonorgestrel (LNG) EC decreases the risk of pregnancy from 8% to 1% to 2% after a single episode of unprotected intercourse (**Table 4**).[40]

LNG is a progestin-only EC pill that is taken orally as soon as possible, within a 72-hour window following sexual intercourse, although some studies suggest moderate efficacy up to 120 hours postcoitus.[41–44] LNG EC is sold in the United States as Plan B One-Step (1.5 mg) as a single dose and is sold over the counter without restrictions by age or gender. It is sold under several generic labels, including Take Action, My Way, AfterPill (available only online), Aftera, and Option 2. For many people, this method is known as Plan B (the original morning-after pill sold as two doses taken 12 hours apart) or the "morning-after pill." It costs about $50 for brand name and about

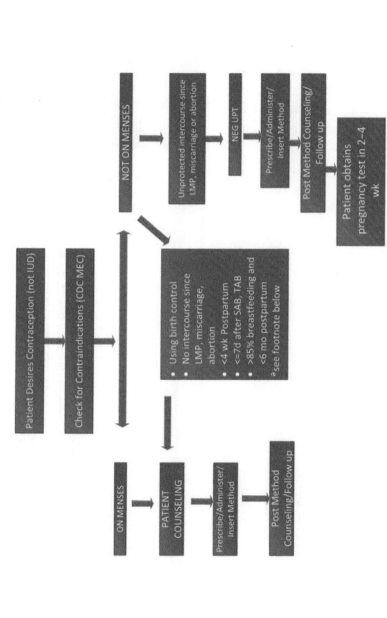

Fig. 2. Contraception flow chart (not IUD). [a] If a woman does not meet any of these criteria, then the health care provider cannot be reasonably sure that she is not pregnant, even with a pregnancy test. On the basis of clinical judgement, the health care provider may consider the addition of a urine pregnancy test; however, they should be aware of the limitations, including accuracy of the test relative to the time of last sexual intercourse, recent delivery, or spontaneous or induced abortion. Routine pregnancy testing for every woman is not necessary.[10] LMP, last menstrual period; Neg UPT, negative urine pregnancy test; SAB, spontaneous abortion or early pregnancy loss; TAB, therapeutic abortion, induced abortion or termination of pregnancy.

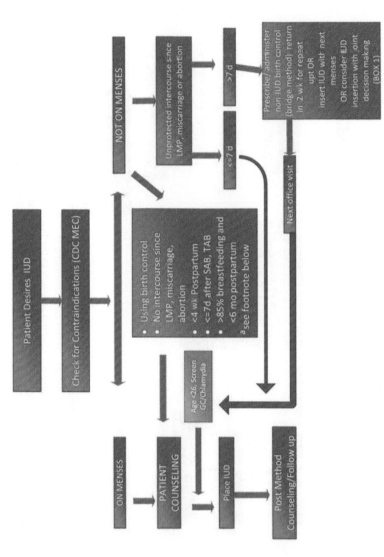

Fig. 3. Contraception flow chart IUD. [a] If a woman does not meet any of these criteria, then the health care provider cannot be reasonably sure that she is not pregnant, even with a pregnancy test. On the basis of clinical judgement, the health care provider may consider the addition of a urine pregnancy test; however, they should be aware of the limitations, including accuracy of the test relative to the time of last sexual intercourse, recent delivery, or spontaneous or induced abortion. Routine pregnancy testing for every woman is not necessary.[10] LMP, last menstrual period; GC, gonorrhea; SAB, spontaneous abortion or early pregnancy loss; TAB, therapeutic abortion.

Table 2
LNG-containing IUDs in the United States and Copper T

Brand Name	Mirena	Liletta	Skyla	Kyleena	Paragard
Dosage, mg	52	52	13.5	19.5	No hormone
Duration of use/Food and Drug Administration labeling, y	5 Off label 7 y[20-39]	4	3	5	10 y Off label 12 y[18,19]
Intrauterine device size, mm	32 × 32	32 × 32	30 × 28	30 × 28	32 × 36
Insertion tube diameter, mm	4.4	4.8	3.8	3.8	4.38
Thread color	Brown	Blue	Brown	Blue	White

Table 3
Contraceptive options available in the United States

Method	Mechanism of Action	Administration	Effectiveness Perfect/Typical Use, %	Advantages	Common Side Effects/ Disadvantages
Nexplanon	Inhibits ovulation, thickens cervical mucous	4-cm rod inserted 6–10 cm proximal to the medial epicondyle and 3.5 cm inferior to the groove between the biceps and triceps (typically in the nondominant arm)	99/99	Effective 3–5 y (limited data in those with BMI >30), discrete, nothing to do once it is placed, rapid return to fertility	Health care provider must insert and remove Irregular bleeding is common but not harmful
Progesterone IUD	Renders endometrium unfavorable because of inflammatory response, thickens cervical mucous	T-shaped device inserted in the uterus/fundus; small string hangs from cervix for removal (but is cut short or placed inside cervix for bothersome symptoms or discretion)	>99/>99	Lasts 3–7 y depending on method (see **Table 5**) Lighter periods, many with amenorrhea, reduced cramps, rapid return to fertility	Irregular bleeding Discomfort with insertion Rare expulsion (<1/100) and perforation (<1/1000)
Copper T IUD	Renders endometrium unfavorable because of inflammatory response	Same as progesterone IUD Different insertor device	>99/>99	Lasts 12 y Nonhormonal Rapid return to fertility Can also be used within 5 d of intercourse for emergency contraception	Same as progesterone IUD Associated with longer and heavier periods during the first months after insertion, but not harmful

Medroxyprogesterone acetate	Inhibits ovulation, thickens cervical mucous	Intramuscular injection (typically arm or buttock) every 11–15 wk	99/97	Every 3 mo dosing Many women are amenorrheic or have reduced periods after second dose Top-tier contraceptive choice for women with epilepsy/seizure disorders because it may reduce seizure frequency	Irregular bleeding is common but not harmful, prolonged anovulation after cessation (1–4 mo on average)
Transdermal patch	Prevents ovulation by suppressing hypothalamic and subsequently pituitary hormone release	Patch placed on skin (not on breasts) weekly for 3 wk and then 1 patch-free wk Most experts discourage extended/continuous use for consideration of elevated estrogen levels associated with this method	99/92 May be more effective than pills	Improves acne and dysmenorrhea, protects against ovarian/ endometrial cancer, benign breast disease Used for treating PMS/PMDD, polycystic ovarian disease, endometriosis, menstrual migraines Weekly use	Nausea, breast tenderness, irregular bleeding, patch detachment and irritation May not be as effective in obese patients May be associated with higher risk of thromboembolic events
Contraceptive ring	Same as patch	Small ring placed by patient intravaginally for 3 wk and it is removed for 1 week Or ring can be used for 1 mo for menstrual suppression/continuous use	99/92 May be more effective than pills	Same as contraceptive patch Monthly use	If bothersome during sex, can remove for up to 3 h Can use empty tampon inserter to push it in the vagina

(continued on next page)

Table 3
(continued)

Method	Mechanism of Action	Administration	Effectiveness Perfect/Typical Use, %	Advantages	Common Side Effects/ Disadvantages
Combined oral contraceptive pills	Same as patch and ring	One pill daily, can use cyclically to have menses every month, extended use to have menses every 3 mo or continuously to suppress menses	99/92	Same as patch and ring Daily use	Nausea, breast tenderness, irregular bleeding
Progesterone-only pills (mini pill)	Same as medroxyprogesterone acetate	One pill daily	99/90–97	Can be used while breastfeeding Option for those who cannot use estrogen contraceptive methods	Must be taken at the same time each day
Female/male sterilization	Permanent sterilization to block, cut, or remove the tubes	Requires surgery Fallopian tubes are cut, tied, or removed Vas deferens are cut	99	Salpingectomy reduces ovarian cancer Definitive option	Requires surgery Does not offer improvement in menstrual cycles or ovulation suppression
Condoms (male)	Serves as a barrier to sperm	Placed before sexual intercourse	98/85	Also protects against STIs	Latex allergy Often used incorrectly and inconsistently
Condoms (female)	Same as male condom	Sheaths, or linings, that fit loosely inside a woman's vagina, made of thin, transparent, soft plastic film	90/79	Also protects against STIs	Same as male condom

Diaphragm, sponges, and caps	Covers the cervix to serve as a barrier to sperm	Dome-shaped cup	>82	Also protects against STIs Can be put in before sex and left in for 24 h Nonhormonal method	Needs to be used with spermicide Prescription and health care provider visit required to obtain
Spermicide	Inserted into vagina where it immobilizes and kills sperm	Creams, foams, gels, films, and suppositories	72	No prescription needed Can purchase at local store	Low efficacy Should be combined with additional method Needs to be used with every sexual act
Lactational amenorrhea	New breastfeeding mothers	Effective at preventing pregnancy if: (1) <6 mo since the baby was born (2) baby is solely nursing, more than 85% of the time AND (3) amenorrhoeic	99/98	A temporary family planning method based on the natural effect of breastfeeding on fertility	Short interval option Requires consistent breastfeeding
Various tracking methods: basal body temperature, standard days tracking, 2-d method, symptothermal method	Women track their fertile periods by monitoring temperature, mucous, changes in cervix	Women abstain from unprotected vaginal intercourse during fertile days	99/75–98 depending on method	Nonhormonal method	Requires careful and correct monitoring, is difficult if recent or current vaginal infection Requires partner cooperation

Abbreviations: BMI, body mass index; PMDD, premenstrual dysphoric disorder; PMS, premenstrual syndrome; STI, sexually transmitted infection.

Table 4
Emergency contraception

	Copper IUD	Ulipristal Acetate (ELLA)	Levonorgestrel
Efficacy	Most effective	Not as effective as copper IUD, but most effective EC method	Less effective than copper IUD or ulipristal
Timing	Within 5 d after unprotected intercourse (120 h)	Within 5 d after unprotected intercourse (120 h)	Within 3 d after unprotected intercourse (72 h), although may still have efficacy up to 120 h
Available over the counter	No	No	Yes
Timing of birth control after use	Can leave in place for continued use for up to 12 y	Wait 5 d	Immediately (quick start)
Dose	Needs insertion by medical provider	30 mg, single dose	1.5 mg, one dose
BMI	No decrease in efficacy by BMI	Decrease in efficacy for BMI ≥30	Decrease in efficacy for BMI ≥25

Abbreviation: BMI, body mass index.

$40 for generic versions. There are lower cost LNG online options, which cost $20 plus $5 shipping. However, this method is less effective than other EC options (ulipristal acetate [UPA] and copper IUD), particularly for women who are obese or overweight.[44]

UPA, a newer, more effective EC pill, is an antiprogestin sold in the United States as Ella (30 mg). Like LNG EC, it should be taken as soon as possible after unprotected intercourse, but does remain effective for up to 120 hours following intercourse.[44,45]

UPA has been approved by the Food and Drug Administration for use as long as 120 hours after intercourse. It is more expensive than LNG, requires prescription for all ages, and is approved for women who seek an option beyond 72 hours. This method has been shown to be more efficacious for overweight and obese women than LNG EC.[46] Unlike LNG EC, UPA is only available with prescription and is often not immediately available in many pharmacies in the United States. In some states, pharmacists are able to furnish under protocol or prescribe EC, but in most states, a patient must obtain a prescription from a provider. UPA can also be purchased online for about $70, which includes consultation with a physician and shipping. Patients using UPA EC are advised to wait 5 days after use before starting an ongoing progestin-containing hormonal contraceptive method.

The premier form of EC is the copper IUD. It should be inserted within 5 days after unprotected intercourse. It is the most effective EC method, can be retained for effective long-term contraception, and its efficacy is not diminished by patient's weight. One limitation is that the use of the copper IUD does require a timely office visit and a provider to insert the device.

All EC options are important and underused methods to reduce unintended pregnancy. It is one of the key tools in the armamentarium for women not using reliable contraception, between their contraceptive methods, and for those forgetting dosing of their current method. Additionally, it is a key option to remember for patients who are victims of rape or sexual assault.

Special Considerations

Postpartum contraception

After childbirth, the recommended period before attempting the next pregnancy is 18 to 24 months.[47] Despite this recommendation, 33% of unintended pregnancies are within 18 months of a previous live birth.[48] Interpregnancy intervals less than 18 months are associated with adverse outcomes including low-birth-weight infant, preterm delivery, intrauterine fetal demise, and early neonatal demise.[49,50] Since the World Health Organization recommendation to promote spacing of interval pregnancies to 24 months, there has been some in-depth analysis suggesting that the risks associated with short interpregnancy intervals may be confounded by such factors as maternal characteristics and socioeconomic status. Future studies on interpregnancy intervals, with better control for confounding factors, particularly in the United States, will shed a greater light on this issue. Postpartum contraception is important to initiate before resuming sexual activity. Approximately 50% of women have resumed intercourse by 6 weeks after delivery.[51,52] Adolescents are a particularly high-risk group for closely spaced pregnancy because studies have demonstrated that more than 50% of postpartum teenagers had intercourse before starting any form of birth control.[53] When considering the timing of postpartum contraception, it is important to consider when ovulation resumes for the postpartum patient. For women who are fully breastfeeding, ovulation occurs for 20% by 12 weeks; for those not fully breastfeeding, ovulation resumes for about 50% by 6 weeks; and for those who are not breastfeeding, ovulation resumes at 4 weeks.[51] Prompt initiation of contraception after childbirth is critical to prevent unplanned and closely spaced pregnancies. Ultimately postpartum contraception reduces the likelihood of unintended pregnancy and improves the health of mothers and babies by lengthening birth intervals. Contraceptive plans should optimally be discussed at prenatal care visits. Counseling and a full range of contraceptive options should be available at the time of delivery and/or before discharge from the hospital. When counseling women about postpartum contraceptive options, it is helpful to consider that postpartum women have reported some of the most important qualities in a contraceptive method are: ease of use, the absence of a need for monthly pharmacy trips, long-term protection, and safety during breastfeeding (**Table 5**).[54]

Postpartum contraception has been redefined, most specifically for LARCs, as immediate postpartum contraception (before discharge from the hospital) or "delayed" or "interval" contraception, which is generally defined as placement at the postpartum visit. Immediate contraceptive administration is one important modality that provides effective, long-term birth control without repeated trips to the pharmacy or an uncomfortable follow-up visit when they return at 6 to 8 weeks. In the United States, more than 40% of women do not return for a postpartum visit. To minimize barriers to effective contraception in the United States, IUDs are increasingly being placed after delivery of baby and placenta, and implants are being placed before patients are discharged home from the hospital.

To promote and optimize postpartum contraception and access, the American College of Obstetricians and Gynecologists has developed a LARC program (https://www.acog.org/About-ACOG/ACOG-Departments/Long-Acting-Reversible-Contraception) and Postpartum Contraceptive Access Initiative (https://pcainitiative.acog.org/) to help promote and prepare obstetrician-gynecologists and other health care providers to offer the full range of contraceptive methods to women after delivery through comprehensive, individualized training.

Contraception for women with intellectual and developmental disabilities

When caring for people with intellectual or developmental disabilities, it is important to remember that they are sexual beings and may have the same contraceptive needs as those without challenges. Thus, education about reproductive health, contraceptive options, and special circumstances for administering contraception is important when treating these patients. Health care providers should be aware that patients with a physical or developmental disability, or both, are at higher risk of sexual assault compared with their peers without special needs. For health care providers who care for medically complex patients, the importance of contraception to prevent unintended pregnancy should be emphasized. Health care providers may reference the CDC US MEC for contraceptive use for guidance caring for those with complex medical conditions.[45] Expert consultation should be requested if questions remain regarding the safest choices for contraception.

Reproductive Coercion and Birth Control Sabotage

For all people, selecting contraception is a "highly preference-sensitive decision" and providers should encourage patient-centered shared decision-making. This is particularly relevant in communities with concentrated social disadvantage where histories of reproductive injustice, structural inequalities, and systemic racism continue to influence access to health care and perceptions of contraception.[55]

Violence against women is a well-recognized factor in increasing women's risk for unintended pregnancies. Reproductive coercion is a form of intimate partner violence where women experience pressure from their partners to become pregnant, including condom manipulation and contraceptive sabotage, and has been closely associated

Table 5
Postpartum contraception

Condition		OCPs	Progestin-Only Method	Medroxyprogesterone Acetate	Implant	LNG-IUD	Copper IUD
Postpartum	<21 d	4	1	1	1		
	21–42 d						
	(a) With no other risk factors for VTE	3	1	1	1		
	(b) Without other risk factors for VTE	2	1	1	1		
	>42 d	1	1	1	1		
Postpartum (in breastfeeding or nonbreastfeeding women including post cesarean section)	(a) <10 min after delivery of the placenta					2	1
	(b) 10 min after delivery of placenta to <4 wk					2	2
	(c) ≥4 wk					1	1
	(d) Puerperal sepsis						
Breastfeeding	(a) <1 mo postpartum	3	2	2	2		
	(b) 1 mo or more postpartum	2	1		1		

Abbreviations: **1**, no restriction (method can be used); **2**, advantages generally outweigh theoretic or proven risks; **3**, theoretic or proven risks usually outweigh the advantages; **4**, unacceptable health risk (method not to be used); OCP, oral contraceptive pill; VTE, venous thromboembolism.

Adapted from Centers for Disease Control and Prevention (CDC). US Medical Eligibility Criteria (US MEC) for contraceptive use, 2016. Available at: https://www.cdc.gov/reproductivehealth/contraception/mmwr/mec/summary.html. Accessed April 4, 2019.

with unintended pregnancy. Miller and colleagues[56] surveyed almost 1300 women seeking care at Northern California family planning clinics and found more than 50% of the women reported lifetime prevalence of physical or sexual partner violence, 19% reported ever experiencing pressure to get pregnant, and 15% reported contraceptive sabotage, all associated with unintended pregnancy. The CDC 2010 National Intimate Partner and Sexual Violence Survey estimates that 8.6% of women in the United States have experienced reproductive coercion in their intimate relationships.[57] Intimate partner violence, and reproductive coercion specifically, may influence women's decision-making, and providers should be aware of their role in supporting women who have been exposed to such abuse. LARCs can serve as an ideal stealth contraceptive method to reduce unintended pregnancy in this population. Many women choose a hormonal IUD with the strings cut short; a progestin implant, which is often discrete; or even a nonhormonal IUD in circumstances where partners are tracking their periods. Thus, LARCs can serve as a harm-reduction strategy to reduce risk for an unwanted pregnancy and as a means of empowering women. A randomized trial of a reproductive coercion intervention in family planning clinics demonstrated increased self-efficacy to enact harm-reduction strategies and reduced reproductive coercion a year later.[58] Providers can offer education about reproductive coercion and offer LARC as one way to discretely prevent pregnancy.

SUMMARY

The health care provider serves as an important touch point for helping women plan and prevent their pregnancies. Contraception counseling should be addressed at every health care visit during the reproductive years, including prenatal visits. A health care provider can ask just one key question at each well-woman visit: Are you interested in getting pregnant this year? Health care providers are ideally poised to educate patients on contraceptive options, to assist in making joint decisions on methods that address her unique phase in life, and to prescribe or place methods in a single visit to reduce barriers to obtaining contraception. Contraception improves the overall health of women and can provide unique opportunities for empowerment during various chapters of woman's life. Anticipatory guidance and dispelling misinformation continue to be paramount to promoting acceptance and retention of various contraceptive methods. Ongoing and future research into contraception arenas, such as optimizing postpartum contraception, identifying strategies and methods that minimize side effects, and approaches that improve access to contraception in the United States and globally, will all help women and their families' live healthier, longer, and happier lives.

REFERENCES

1. Contraceptive use in the US. Available at: https://www.guttmacher.org/united-states/contraception. Accessed December 5, 2018.

2. Trussell J. Contraceptive failure in the United States. Contraception 2011;83(5): 397–404.

3. Finer LB, Zolna MR. Declines in unintended pregnancy in the United States, 2008–2011. N Engl J Med 2016;374:843–52.

4. Sonfield A, Hasstedt K, Gold R. Moving forward: family planning in the era of health reform. New York: Guttmacher Institute; 2014. Available at: https://www.guttmacher.org/report/moving-forward-family-planning-era-health-reform. Accessed December 5, 2018.

5. Trussell J, Guthrie KA. Choosing a contraceptive: efficacy, safety, and personal considerations. In: Hatcher RA, et al, editors. Contraceptive technology. 20th revised edition. New York: Ardent Media; 2011. p. 45–74.

6. Madden T, Mullersman JL, Omkig KJ, et al. Structured contraceptive counseling program provided by the Contraceptive CHOICE Project. Contraception 2013; 88(2):243–9.

7. Lee JK, Parisi SM, Akers AY, et al. The impact of contraception counseling in primary care on contraceptive use. J Gen Intern Med 2011;26(7):731–6.

8. Atrash HK, Johnson K, Adams M, et al. Preconception care for improving perinatal outcomes the time to act. Matern Child Health J 2006;10(5 Suppl):S3–11.

9. World Health Organization. Medical eligibility criteria for contraceptive use. 4th edition 2010. Geneva (Switzerland). Available at: https://www.cdc.gov/reproductivehealth/unintendedpregnancy/pdf/legal_summary-chart_english_final_tag508.pdf. Accessed December 5, 2018.

10. Centers for Disease Control and Prevention. United States selected practice recommendations for contraceptive use. MMWR Morb Mortal Wkly Rep 2013; 62(RR-5):1–60. Available at: https://www.cdc.gov/reproductivehealth/contraception/mmwr/spr/summary.html. Accessed December 5, 2018.

11. Wilson JG, Brent RL. Are female sex hormones teratogenic? Am J Obstet Gynecol 1981;141(5):567–80.

12. Westhoff C, Heartwell S, Edwards S, et al. Initiation of oral contraceptives using a quick start compared with a conventional start: a randomized controlled trial. Obstet Gynecol 2007;109(6):1270–6.

13. Westhoff C, Osborne LM, Schafer JE, et al. Bleeding patters after immediate initiation of an oral compared with vaginal hormonal contraceptive. Obstet Gynecol 2005;106(1):89–96.

14. Murthy AS, Crenin MD, Harwood B, et al. Same-day initiation of the transdermal hormonal delivery system (contraceptive patch) versus traditional initiation methods. Contraception 2005;72(5):333–6.

15. Adolescents and long-acting reversible contraception: implants and intrauterine devices. Committee Opinion No. 539. American College of Obstetricians and Gynecologists. Obstet Gynecol 2012;120:983–8.

16. Women's preventative service initiative. Available at: https://www.womenspreventivehealth.org/. Accessed December 5, 2018.

17. Kavanaugh ML, Jerman J. Contraceptive method use in the United States: trends and characteristics between 2008 and 2014. Contraception 2018;97(1):14–21.

18. United Nations Development Programme, United Nations Population Fund, World Health Organization, World Bank, Special Programme of Research, Development and Research Training in Human Reproduction. Long-term reversible contraception: twelve years of experience with the TCu380A and TCu220C. Contraception 1997;56:341–52.

19. Ali M, Akin A, Bahamondes L, et al. Extended use up to 5 years of the etonogestrel-releasing subdermal contraceptive implant: comparison to levonorgestrel-releasing subdermal implant. Hum Reprod 2016;31:2491–8.

20. Rowe P, Farley T, Peregoudov A, et al, IUD Research Group of the UNDP/UNFPA/WHO/World Bank Special Programme of Research; Development and Research Training in Human Reproduction. Safety and efficacy in parous women of a 52-mg levonorgestrel-medicated intrauterine device: a 7-year randomized comparative study with the TCu380A. Contraception 2016;93:498–506.

21. McNicholas C, Swor E, Wan L, et al. Prolonged use of the etonogestrel implant and levonorgestrel intrauterine device: 2 years beyond Food and Drug Administration-approved duration. Am J Obstet Gynecol 2017;216:586.e1-e6.

22. Faúndes A, Alvarez F, Díaz J. A Latin American experience with levonorgestrel IUD. Ann Med 1993;25:149–53.

23. Ronnerdag M, Odlind V. Health effects of long-term use of the intrauterine levonorgestrel releasing system. A follow-up study over 12 years of continuous use. Acta Obstet Gynecol Scand 1999;78:716–21.

24. Hidalgo MM, Hidalgo-Regina C, Bahamondes MV, et al. Serum levonorgestrel levels and endometrial thickness during extended use of the levonorgestrel-releasing intrauterine system. Contraception 2009;80:84–9.

25. Madden T, Proehl S, Allsworth JE, et al. Naprosyn or estradiol for bleeding and spotting with the levonorgestrel intrauterine system: a randomized control trial. Am J Obstet Gynecol 2012;206:129.e1-8.

26. Hou MY, McNicholas C, Creinin MD. Combined oral contraceptive treatment for bleeding complaints with the etonogestrel contraceptive implant: a randomised controlled trial. Eur J Contracept Reprod Health Care 2016;21(5):361–6.

27. Mansour D, Bahamondes L, Critchley H, et al. The management of unacceptable bleeding patterns in etonorgestrel-releasing contraceptive implant users. Contraception 2011;83:202–10.

28. Guiahi M, McBride M, Sheeder J, et al. Short-term treatment of bothersome bleeding for etonorgestrel implant users using a 14-day oral contraceptive pill regimen: a randomized controlled trial. Obstet Gynecol 2015;126:508–13.

29. Weisberg E, Hickey M, Palmer D, et al. A randomized controlled trial of treatment options for troublesome uterine bleeding in Implanon users. Hum Reprod 2009; 24:1852–61.

30. Bonny AE, Ziegler J, Harvey R, et al. Weight gain in obese and nonobese adolescent girls initiating depot medroxyprogesterone, oral contraceptive pills, or no hormonal contraceptive method. Arch Pediatr Adolesc Med 2006;160(1):40–5.

31. Harel Z, Johnson CC, Gold MA, et al. Recovery of bone mineral density in adolescents following the use of depot medroxyprogesterone acetate contraceptive injections. Contraception 2010;81(4):L281–91.

32. Scholes D, LaCroix AZ, Ichikawa Le, et al. Change in bone mineral density among adolescent women using and discontinuing depot medroxyprogesterone acetate contraception. Arch Pediatr Adolesc Med 2005;159(2):139–44.

33. Cromer BA, Scholes D, Berenson A, et al. Depo medroxyprogesterone acetate and bone mineral density in adolescents -the black box warning: a position paper of the society for adolescent medicine. J Adolesc Health 2006;39(2):296–301.

34. Committee on Adolescent Health Care and Committee on Gynecologic Practice. ACOG committee opinion no. 415: depot medroxyprogesterone acetate and bone effects. Obstet Gynecol 2008;112(3):727–30.

35. Daniels K, Mosher WD, Jones J. Contraceptive methods women have ever used: United States, 1982–2010. Natl Health Stat Report 2013;(62):1–15.

36. Davis AR, Pack AM, Dennis A. Contraception for women with epilepsy. In: Allen RH, Cwiak CA, editors. Contraception for the medically challenging patient. New York: Springer Science+Business Media; 2014. p. 135–46.

37. Jick SS, Hagberg KW, Hernandez R, et al. Postmarketing studies of ORTHOEVRA and levonorgestrel oral contraceptives containing hormone contraceptives with 30 mcg of ethinyl estradiol in relation to nonfatal venous thromboembolism. Contraception 2010;81(1):16–21.

38. Collaborative Group on Epidemiological Studies of Ovarian Cancer. Ovarian cancer and oral contraceptives: collaborative reanalysis of data from 45 epidemiological studies including 23,257 women with ovarian cancer and 87,303 controls. Lancet 2008;371:303–14.

39. Kaunitz AM. Noncontraceptive health benefits of oral contraceptives. Rev Endocr Metab Disord 2002;3(3):277–83.

40. Randomized controlled trial of levonorgestrel verses Yuzpe regimen of combined oral contraceptives for emergency contraception. Task Force on Postovulatory Methods of Fertility Regulation. Lancet 1998;352:428–33.

41. Glasier AF, Cameron ST, Fine PM, et al. Ulipristal acetate versus levonorgestrel for emergency contraception: a randomised non-inferiority trial and meta-analysis. Lancet 2010;375(9714):555–62.

42. Piaggio G, Kapp N, von Hertzen H. Effect on pregnancy rates of the delay in the administration of levonorgestrel for emergency contraception: a combined analysis of four WHO trials. Contraception 2011;84(1):35–9, 13.

43. Curtis KM, Jatlaoui TC, Tepper NK, et al. U.S. selected practice recommendations for contraceptive use, 2016. MMWR Recomm Rep 2016;65(4):1–66, 14.

44. Faculty of Sexual & Reproductive Healthcare. Emergency contraception March 2017 (updated December 2017). London: Faculty of Sexual & Reproductive Healthcare; 2017. p. 1–52.

45. Curtis KM, Tepper NK, Jatlaoui TC, et al. Medical eligibility criteria for contraceptive use, 2016. MMWR Recomm Rep 2016;65(3):1–103.

46. Praditpan P, Hamouie A, Basaraba CN, et al. Pharmacokinetics of levonorgestrel and ulipristal acetate emergency contraception in women with normal and obese body mass index. Contraception 2017;95(5):464–9.

47. World Health Organization. Report of a WHO technical consultation on birth spacing. Geneva (Switzerland): WHO Press; 2007. WHO/RHR/07.1 World Health Organization; Available at: http://www.who.int/making_pregnancy_safer/documents/birth_spacing05/en/index.html. Accessed: December 5, 2018.

48. Zapata LB, Murtaza S, Whiteman MK, et al. Contraceptive counseling and postpartum contraceptive use. Am J Obstet Gynecol 2015;212(2):171.e1-e8.

49. Cohen R, Sheeder J, Arango N, et al. Twelve-month contraceptive continuation and repeat pregnancy among young mothers choosing postdelivery contraceptive implants or postplacental intrauterine devices. Contraception 2016;93:179–83.

50. Goldthwaite LM, Shaw KA. Immediate postpartum provision of long-acting reversible contraception. Curr Opin Obstet Gynecol 2015;27:460–4.

51. Speroff L, Mishell DR Jr. The postpartum visit: it's time for a change in order to optimally initiate contraception. Contraception 2008;78:90–8.

52. Lewis LN, Doherty DA, Hickey M, et al. Implanon as a contraceptive choice for teenage mothers: a comparison of contraceptive choices, acceptability, and repeat pregnancy. Contraception 2010;81:421–6.

53. Tocce K, Sheeder J, Python J, et al. Long acting reversible contraception in postpartum adolescents: early initiation of etonogestrel implant is superior to IUDs in the outpatient setting. J Pediatr Adolesc Gynecol 2002;25:59–63.

54. Cwiak C, Gellasch T, Zieman M. Peripartum contraceptive attitudes and practices. Contraception 2004;70:383–6.

55. Higgins JA. Celebration meets caution: long acting reversible contraception (LARC)'s boons, potential busts, and the benefits of a reproductive justice approach. Contraception 2014;89(4):237–41.

56. Miller E, Decker MR, Mccauley H, et al. Pregnancy coercion, intimate partner violence and unintended pregnancy. Contraception 2010;81:316–22.
57. Black MC, Basile K, Breiding M, et al. The National Intimate Partner and Sexual Violence Survey (NISVS): 2010 summary report. Atlanta (GA): National Center for Injury Prevention and Control Centers for Disease Control and Prevention; 2011.
58. Miller E, Tancredi DJ, Decker MR, et al. A family planning clinic-based intervention to address reproductive coercion: a cluster randomized controlled trial. Contraception 2016;94(1):58–67.

Optimizing Health
Weight, Exercise, and Nutrition in Pregnancy and Beyond

Elizabeth A. Hoover, MD, Judette M. Louis, MD, MPH*

KEYWORDS

- Obesity • Weight • Exercise • Nutrition • Diet • Pregnancy
- Maternal and perinatal outcomes

KEY POINTS

- Obesity and excessive gestational weight gain are associated with adverse perinatal outcomes.
- Excessive gestational weight gain is associated with postpartum weight retention and obesity, leading to lifelong impacts on maternal health.
- Exercise and nutrition play an important role in reducing excessive gestational weight gain, particularly during pregnancy when women are inherently motivated to make lifestyle modifications.
- Obstetric providers should use the opportunity provided by the interpregnancy period to optimize the health of women at risk.

INTRODUCTION

It is well-established that pregnancy complications provide insight into women's future health risks and have long-term implications for maternal and child health. Hypertensive disorders of pregnancy, gestational diabetes, intrauterine growth restriction, and preterm delivery are indicators of future cardiovascular disease risk and should raise concern for development of worsening health status with future pregnancy and across a woman's life span. The Women's Preventive Services Initiative states that screening for obesity should be a routine part of well-woman health care across the lifespan.[1] Although screening and treating obesity can be challenging, the American College of Obstetricians and Gynecologists (ACOG) has provided a toolkit to assist health care providers with obesity screening, evaluation, and treatment. The ACOG provides recommendations for lifestyle behaviors and recognizes that health care providers play a pivotal role.

Disclosure Statement: The authors have nothing to disclose.
Department of Obstetrics and Gynecology, Division of Maternal Fetal Medicine, University of South Florida, 2 Tampa General Circle, 6th Floor, Tampa, FL 33606, USA
* Corresponding author.
E-mail address: jlouis1@health.usf.edu

Excessive weight gain during pregnancy or retention of the weight gained in pregnancy increases women's risk for developing obesity and the correlated chronic morbidity.[2] Obesity has been associated with adverse perinatal outcomes and is a risk factor for long-term cardiovascular disease and metabolic syndrome.[3] In a culture in which reproductive-age women often only seek medical care during pregnancy, pregnancy and the postpartum period provides a unique opportunity to discuss women's health beyond pregnancy, emphasize the importance of interconception care, and implement appropriate primary and secondary prevention strategies for women at risk of chronic disease.[2] (See Dr. Diana E. Ramos' article, "Preconception Health: Changing the Paradigm on Well-Woman Health," in this issue.) However, discussion is frequently focused on the current pregnancy alone or not communicated to women's nonobstetric health providers. This precludes planning for the future health of the woman.

It is the author's aim to review the impact of gestational weight gain, postpartum weight retention, and obesity on pregnancy and lifelong maternal health. The role of exercise and nutrition in prevention of excessive gestational weight gain, postpartum weight retention, and obesity in pregnancy and beyond is discussed.

Gestational Weight Gain

In 2009, the Institute of Medicine (IOM) revised the guidelines for gestational weight gain. Two major modifications included the use of the World Health Organization body mass index (BMI) categories as a measure of prepregnancy weight and specific ranges of recommended weight gain for obese women. According to the 2009 IOM guidelines, underweight women (BMI <18.5 kg/m^2) are recommended a gestational weight gain of 28 to 40 pounds. For women of normal weight (BMI 18.5 kg/m^2–24.9 kg/m^2), gestational weight gain should aim between 25 to 35 pounds. Overweight women (BMI 25 kg/m^2–29.9 kg/m^2) are recommended to gain between 15 to 25 pounds, whereas obese women (BMI $\geq$30 kg/m^2) should limit weight gain to 11 to 20 pounds.[4] However, the 2009 IOM recommendations are limited because the term obesity does not account for the continuum of BMI greater than or equal to 30 kg/m^2.[3] In particular, there are no specific recommendations for women with morbid obesity.

Weight gain in excess of the IOM guidelines has been termed excessive gestational weight gain. Despite the clear guidelines, it is estimated that 48% of all women of reproductive-age exceed the recommended weight gain in pregnancy.[5] Excessive gestational weight gain has been associated with an increased risk of pregnancy complications, including gestational diabetes, hypertensive disorders of pregnancy, and cesarean delivery, regardless of the prepregnancy BMI.[4] Beyond the acute risks to the pregnancy, there are also future implications. Retention of excessive gestational weight increases the probability of entering the next pregnancy as obese or overweight. These women can then be caught in a perpetually exacerbated cycle of excessive gestational weight gain and weight retention, entering each subsequent pregnancy at a higher weight than previous pregnancies. These cycles of excessive weight gain and high weight retention predispose women to future obesity.

Postpartum Weight Retention

Weight retention, the difference between postpartum weight and prepregnancy weight, following pregnancy is of equal concern. Many women of normal weight before pregnancy may gain excessive gestational weight and have increased difficulty losing this weight following pregnancy.[6] The degree of the weight retained postpartum is highly variable between women (and often depends on the amount of gestational weight gain).[5] Women with excess gestational weight gain retain the most weight postpartum. Women who are overweight and obese in the preconception period are more likely to experience postpartum weight retention. Past studies indicated that only 11% of overweight and obese pregnant women return to their preconception weight within 5 years postpartum.[5]

An ideal length of time women should return to prepregnancy weight postpartum has not been established; however, recommendations have been made to aim for 6 months to 1 year postpartum.[7] In one report, women losing pregnancy weight by 6 months postpartum were only 2.4 kg heavier on investigation 10 years later compared with 8.3 kg in those who did not return to prepregnancy weight within 6 months following delivery.[8]

Excessive Weight Gain, Weight Retention, and Future Health

Excessive weight gain during pregnancy is the strongest risk factor for postpartum weight retention. With gestational weight gain of 16 kg or more during pregnancy, women were 2.5 times more likely to retain that weight at 1 year postpartum.[5] This weight retention predisposes woman to future obesity.

In addition to the retained weight and subsequent obesity, excessive gestational weight gain has been associated with subsequent development of type 2 diabetes mellitus. Women who exceeded the IOM guidelines for gestational weight gain, when compared with women with appropriate weight gain, were 47% more likely to experience diabetes mellitus at 21 years postpartum. This association was mediated by the woman's current BMI but not any other clinical or demographic characteristics. After a women is diagnosed with gestational diabetes, every 1 pound per week additional increase in weight gain is associated with a 36% to 83% increase in pregnancy-related hypertension.[5]

Other studies have demonstrated an association between excessive gestational weight gain and future obesity, diabetes, and metabolic syndrome. These are all chronic diseases that have been identified as risk factors for future cardiovascular disease, potentially increasing the morbidity and mortality among these women. For women with excessive gestational weight gain and weight retention, counseling regarding the short-term and long-term implications of the weight gain should be included as part of the postpartum, interpregnancy, or well-woman care visits.

OBESITY: IMPLICATIONS FOR PREGNANCY

Obesity among reproductive-age women is prevalent and increasing.[6] Greater than one-third of reproductive-age women are currently considered obese (BMI ≥ 30 kg/m^2), with 10% of these women meeting criteria for morbid obesity (BMI ≥ 40 kg/m^2). Obesity among this population has been associated with adverse perinatal outcomes and carries short-term and long-term implications for maternal and child health. It is imperative that health care providers caring for women of reproductive-age appreciate the importance of obesity as a risk factor for perinatal and long-term maternal health complications and tailor their care accordingly.[3] The following obesity-associated risks should be reviewed with all women of reproductive-age.

Antepartum Considerations

Fetal complications
Obesity is associated with fetal complications, including spontaneous abortion, fetal anomalies, fetal macrosomia, intrauterine growth restriction, and intrauterine fetal demise.[3] The association between increasing obesity and fetal anomalies has been

well-demonstrated in many studies.[9] These anomalies can be severe and include cardiac, nervous system, and limb abnormalities. The etiologic factors of spontaneous abortion and congenital anomalies in this population remain unknown; however, metabolic changes, undiagnosed diabetes, and nutritional deficiencies have been proposed as possible causes.[3]

Fetal growth in the setting of maternal obesity can be compromised, resulting in intrauterine growth restriction and associated complications such as indicated preterm delivery. However, obesity is also associated with large-for-gestational-age fetuses, even after controlling for maternal diabetes.[3] This is concerning because 50% of large for gestational age infants will develop obesity and metabolic syndrome between the ages of 6 and 11 years.[10]

Infants born from pregnancies complicated by diabetes are at risk for fetal macrosomia, increased adiposity, shoulder dystocia, birth injury, and cesarean delivery. These infants are at higher risk of obesity themselves by age 2 years and development of type 2 diabetes as adults.[5]

Prenatal screening

The obese gravida faces challenges in prenatal diagnosis. Suboptimal ultrasound visualization due to obesity has been reported to negatively affect detection of fetal anomalies by as much as 30%.

Genetic screening can also be significantly limited by maternal obesity. The first trimester screen may be limited by an inability to obtain nuchal translucency measurement via ultrasound. The quadruple serum screen for aneuploidy is known to have an increased false-positive rate in women with obesity secondary to the use of a standard weight correction by laboratories that does not exceed 270 pounds. Maternal serum cell-free DNA testing, a more contemporary screening test for aneuploidy, is limited because fetal fraction decreases as maternal weight increases. If fetal fraction is less than 4%, the noninvasive prenatal screening is unable to provide results. Diagnostic procedures, such as amniocentesis or chorionic villus sampling, are technically more difficult with increased abdominal adiposity.[3] It is imperative to counsel overweight and obese women entering pregnancy about the increased risk of fetal malformations, as well as the difficulty in detecting those abnormalities due to obesity.

Maternal health

Women with obesity are more likely to enter pregnancy with underlying medical comorbidities, including chronic hypertension, type 2 diabetes, obstructive sleep apnea, liver and gallbladder disease, musculoskeletal pain, and mood disorders. These medical comorbidities should ideally be well-controlled before achieving pregnancy. Medications should be reviewed and altered, if indicated, to prevent teratogenic fetal effects. Thus, obese women and, in particular, women with comorbid conditions, will benefit from preconceptional counseling and health optimization in the interpregnancy period.[3]

Once pregnant, obese gravida are at increased risk for obstetric complications. Compared with normal weight women, they are 3 to 10 times more likely to develop hypertensive disorders of pregnancy, including gestational hypertension and preeclampsia.[6,9] Low-dose aspirin should be considered for women at increased risk of hypertensive disorders of pregnancy, with obesity being considered a moderate risk factor.[1] Use of a proper size arm cuff to measure blood pressure should be ensured. If an appropriate size arm cuff is not available, an arm cuff should be placed on the wrist, and the patient's wrist should be held at or above the level of the heart.[3]

On entering pregnancy, all women with obesity should be considered for evaluation for undiagnosed pregestational diabetes.[3] Glucose screening should be repeated in the second trimester due to the increased risk for development of gestational diabetes in this population.[1,6]

Peripartum Considerations

Labor complications

Obese women are less likely to have spontaneous labor and are more likely to have a postterm pregnancy. This, combined with an increase in underlying comorbidity in this population, results in an increased likelihood of requiring an induction of labor. Increasing BMI is associated with an increased risk of failed induction of labor, operative vaginal delivery, and cesarean delivery.[3,9] Each additional 1 kg/m^2 in BMI increases the risk of cesarean delivery by 4%. Obesity also complicates trial of labor after cesarean delivery, decreasing the rate of successful vaginal delivery. It is currently unknown why obesity contributes to abnormal labor patterns.[3] Should vaginal delivery be feasible, fetuses remain at increased risk for shoulder dystocia and long-term associated neurologic damage, such as brachial plexus injury.[6]

When proceeding to the operating room for cesarean delivery, it is important to consider the possibility of anesthesia-related complications attributed to obesity. The supine position is required for cesarean delivery, and the increased oxygen demands of pregnancy combined with increased burden of weight on the chest wall leads to a high risk of maternal and, subsequently, fetal hypoxemia. Should general anesthesia be required, obstructive sleep apnea or increased adipose tissue in the neck can lead to severe complications with intubation. After placement of epidural or spinal anesthesia, obese women have incurred greater rates of hypotension and fetal heart rate decelerations.[3]

Postoperative concerns

Should cesarean section be required, women with obesity are postoperatively at increased risk for deep venous thrombosis and pulmonary embolism compared with women with normal BMI. This is a major cause of morbidity and mortality among this population. A combination of chemical and mechanical thromboprophylaxis should be considered, if appropriate, in obese patients.[3]

The higher rate of cesarean delivery associated with obesity is further complicated by an increased risk of surgical site infection.[3] Women with obesity should be informed regarding the concern for surgical site infection preoperatively.[9] Evidence-based surgical techniques that include antibiotic prophylaxis, chlorhexidine prep, and reapproximation of subcutaneous tissue should be used to decrease possibility for wound breakdown, and staples should be used to prevent surgical site infection.[3]

INTERVENTIONS TO REDUCE GESTATIONAL WEIGHT GAIN AND WEIGHT RETENTION

Given the interplay between gestational weight gain, obesity, and future health, there has been substantial interest in interventions to reduce gestational weight gain and weight retention during pregnancy and beyond.[11] There is a relationship between menstrual irregularities and obesity. (See Drs Kristen A. Matteson and Kate Zaluski's article, "Menstrual Health as a part of Preventive Health Care," in this issue.) Much of the effort has been focused on lifestyle interventions. A recent meta-analysis of prospective studies found lifestyle interventions to be effective in reducing the proportion of women with excessive gestational weight gain when compared with standard care; however, the difference was modest (61.8% vs 75.0%; odds ratio

0.52, 95% CI 0.40–0.67).[11] The 2 groups did not differ in other outcomes, including birthweight, preeclampsia, gestational diabetes, and cesarean delivery.[11]

Pregnancy and obesity across the lifespan are interrelated. Many reproductive-age women attribute their increasing BMI to pregnancy. Excessive gestational weight gain is independently associated with subsequent obesity across the lifespan. The retained weight postpartum means these women enter the next pregnancy at a higher prepregnancy weight. The gestational weight gain results in a higher BMI category as the woman enters into the next pregnancy. The vicious cycle can continue, resulting in obesity across the lifespan.[5]

Exercise

Historically, pregnant women have been advised to limit physical exertion and exercise secondary to concerns regarding fetal risk. However, promotion of healthy lifestyle and physical exercise during pregnancy is safe for both mother and fetus in otherwise healthy women.[12] Additionally, many women are often motivated to change their lifestyle in pregnancy.[10] The ACOG recommends that all healthy pregnant women follow the Centers for Disease Control and Prevention's activity guidelines and achieve moderate physical activity for 30 minutes or greater nearly every day.[12] Many studies have been undertaken to evaluate the proportion of women engaging in the recommended amount of exercise throughout pregnancy and, although results vary, a study of US women estimated only 15.8% meet this amount of physical activity. Reasons cited for this are diverse, ranging from concern for preterm labor to hesitancy regarding types of appropriate exercise in pregnancy. When entering pregnancy, sedentary women should be encouraged to initiate 15 minutes of exercise every other day and gradually increase to 30 minutes per day most days of the week. Previously active women should be encouraged to maintain their current moderate exercise of at least 30 minutes or greater per day 4 times per week.[13] This level of activity has been shown to help avoid excessive weight gain of pregnancy.[10]

Exercise modality

Aerobic exercise should be recommended to aid cardiovascular fitness. These activities can include walking, jogging, biking, dance, aerobics, and swimming. Health care providers should encourage women to find a form of aerobic exercise that they find enjoyable and sustainable over many years. Women who enjoy particular activities before pregnancy should be encouraged to continue these activities during pregnancy with appropriate modifications as the pregnancy progresses.[13] However, caution regarding the risk of injury from falls, overexertion, Valsalva maneuver, and trauma from contact sports should be given.[10] In all forms of aerobic exercise, warm up and cool down regimens should be incorporated.[13]

In addition to aerobic exercise, strength training is recommended. This form of exercise can occur via Pilates, yoga, weight training, or circuit training. During pregnancy, strength training should be incorporated into a physical fitness regimen once or twice per week on nonconsecutive days. The benefits of strength training include improved posture and core strength, which may relieve musculoskeletal discomfort of pregnancy and improve stamina in labor. Stretching should also be encouraged, although precautions should be given regarding supine positioning in the latter part of pregnancy.[13]

Intensity of exercise

Monitoring of exercise intensity in pregnancy should be encouraged to avoid overexertion. Women can assess this relatively easily via exercising at an intensity that allows one to carry on a conversation. Alternatively, heart rate can be monitored via the use of a fitness tracking device or manually. Maximum heart rate is recommended based on age, corresponding to 60% to 80% of aerobic capacity. In normal-weight women ages 20 to 29 years, a target heart rate of 135 to 150 beats per minute should be obtained; however, in overweight women, this number decreases to 110 to 131 beats per minute.[13]

Benefit of exercise on maternal and neonatal outcomes

It is suggested in a variety of studies that musculoskeletal discomfort associated with pregnancy, such as pelvic, back, or joint pain, can be improved with physical activity.[13] Regular physical exercise in pregnancy helps prevent excessive gestational weight gain and retention of weight after birth. As the previous discussion demonstrates, excessive weight gain in pregnancy and subsequent weight retention complicates pregnancies of all weights and increases the risk of long-term maternal health complications, including development of obesity and cardiovascular disease.[4] In pregnancies affected by gestational diabetes, it has been shown that the addition of physical exertion to dietary modification helps lower blood glucose and reduce insulin requirement. Finally, exercise has been noted to reduce symptoms of depression during pregnancy and the postpartum period. Regarding neonatal outcomes, moderate physical exercise has not been shown to cause decreased infant birthweight or preterm birth.[13]

A significant limitation currently exists in the literature as the above recommendations are intended for women without underlying medical concerns or pregnancy complications. More studies are urgently needed to evaluate the role of exercise in women with underlying medical comorbidities or pregnancy complications. Nevertheless, it is imperative that health care providers emphasize the importance of appropriate physical activity in pregnancy and the subsequent transition of pregnancy habits to lifelong lifestyle modification.[13]

Nutrition

The importance of nutrition in the preconception period and first trimester of pregnancy cannot be understated because this is when organogenesis and other processes critical to fetal development occur. It has been proposed that placental function may be influenced by nutrition during this time, which in turn provides nutrients to the fetus throughout gestation. The absence of adequate maternal nutrition throughout pregnancy can lead to fetal complications, including prematurity, intrauterine growth restriction, fetal anomalies, and infection,[14] as well as a permanent alteration in infant metabolism and subsequent childhood obesity. Low birthweight has been associated with a lower adult BMI but higher risk of metabolic syndrome and central obesity in adulthood compared with normal birthweight. This has been demonstrated by observational studies, including Dutch famine studies from World War II and protein supplementation studies in developing countries.[15]

Maternal nutritional status is influenced early in life, beginning at the time of a woman's own conception and infancy.[15] It has been hypothesized that a poor maternal nutritional status in childhood can lead to poor growth and inadequate pelvic size, ultimately leading to cephalopelvic disproportion and complications with labor. Definitive evidence supporting this association has not yet been demonstrated. One study, however, compared pregnant women of taller physical stature (tall stature serving as a proxy for the presence of adequate childhood nutrition) from industrialized countries not receiving nutritional supplementation during pregnancy to pregnant women in underdeveloped countries receiving nutritional supplementation during pregnancy. This study identified that childhood nutritional status is equally important to maternal nutrition throughout pregnancy in infant birthweight outcomes.[14]

Women of reproductive-age need an adequate supply of proteins, vitamins, and minerals throughout their lives for successful pregnancy outcomes.[15] It is not enough to address maternal nutrition status only during prenatal visits, and women should be educated about nutrition at any opportunity. Furthermore, women entering pregnancy with adequate nutritional status will only require a small amount of additional energy during pregnancy, approximately 240 kcal in the second trimester and 450 kcal in the third trimester. This is because maternal metabolism redirects appropriate amount of nutrients to the placenta and developing fetus [14] Adequate onorgy intake is best assessed by appropriate gestational weight gain.[5]

Women who intend to become pregnant should ensure intake of foods rich in protein, whole grains, fruit, and vegetables in their diets. Micronutrients, such as zinc, calcium, folic acid, vitamin A, iron, and iodine, are critical in early fetal development. Often, women may not realize pregnancy has occurred until this critical developmental period has already passed. Deficiencies in required micronutrients can also exist owing to disease states that result in malabsorption. Supplementation in pregnancy is encouraged to achieve an adequate supply of micronutrients, folate, calcium, and iron.[14]

Breastfeeding

Breastfeeding is affected by obesity, with obese women having an overall decreased rate of breastfeeding, as well as a decreased duration of breastfeeding.[3] Proposed factors responsible for this decrease include prolonged elevation in progesterone levels postdelivery inhibiting lactogenesis, infant admission to neonatal intensive care unit (thus maternal separation postpartum) secondary to labor complications, and challenges with positioning and latching.[9] The benefits of breastfeeding for infants have been well-documented. In recent years there has been more of a focus on the implications for maternal health. Observational studies indicate a decreased risk of diabetes, hypertension, metabolic syndrome, cardiovascular disease, ovarian cancer, and breast cancer among women who breastfed.[7] There is a dose response, with longer durations of breastfeeding showing increased benefit. However, there is insufficient evidence to indicate that breastfeeding decreases weight retention.[7] It is uncertain whether it is breastfeeding that is beneficial to maternal health or if breastfeeding is a marker for another factor that is affecting both maternal health and the ability to breastfeed. Nonetheless, the ACOG recommends exclusive breastfeeding for the first 6 months of life. Anticipatory guidance and counseling should start during the prenatal period to help prepare the mother for the challenges of breastfeeding.[1]

New mothers should be provided reassurance, assistance with positioning and latching by lactation consultants, supplementation when necessary, and postpartum support via telephone follow-up or support groups to facilitate and optimize breastfeeding.[3]

Contraception

Approximately one-third of women become pregnant at a shorter interval than the recommended 18 months, and 45% of all pregnancies are unplanned.[7] Birth spacing and timing is an important tool in the management of women with excessive gestational weight gain, weight retention, or obesity.[7] Counseling about all contraceptive choices should begin during the prenatal period. In women who do not desire any future pregnancies, sterilization can be offered. For women who do not desire sterilization or who plan to have more children, counseling should occur so that women are informed about all of the contraceptive options.[1] The Women's Preventive Services has considered and provided an overview of contraception and empowerment. (See Dr. Nichole Tyson's article, "Reproductive Health: Options, Strategies, and Empowerment of Women," in this issue.) The counseling should take into account obesity, if present, and its contribution to effectiveness of the method chosen.[1] If a decision regarding an alternative contraceptive method is deferred, this can directly contribute to an increased rate of unintended pregnancy and future pregnancy morbidity.[3]

INTERPREGNANCY CARE

Hypertensive disorders of pregnancy, gestational diabetes, intrauterine growth restriction, and preterm delivery are indicators of underlying cardiovascular risk and should raise concern for development of worsening health status with future pregnancy and future cardiovascular disease.[7] In addition, the development of gestational diabetes significantly increases the probability of later developing type 2 diabetes mellitus.[5] Pregnancy and the postpartum period provides an unique opportunity to discuss these risks, emphasize the importance of interconception care, and implement appropriate primary and second prevention strategies for women at risk.[2] Informing women of the lifelong implications of pregnancy complications is an initiative that should be undertaken by all health care providers caring for women of reproductive-age.

The interpregnancy period can be used to optimize maternal health. This time between pregnancies can be transitioned to well-woman care if the woman does not intend future pregnancies. During this time, women can work with their health care providers to optimize their health. This can include weight loss with a goal of reaching prepregnancy weight by 6 to 12 months postpartum.[7] The ideal goal is to enter the next pregnancy at a normal BMI. In addition to nutrition and exercise, the ACOG obesity toolkit provides more resources to help health care providers identify actionable targets. Women with a BMI greater than or equal to 40 kg/m^2 or a BMI greater than or equal to 30 kg/m^2 with obesity-related comorbid conditions may be candidates for bariatric surgery. Weight loss after bariatric surgery has been associated with a reduction in the occurrence of gestational diabetes and hypertensive disorders of pregnancy.[7]

For women who do not desire another pregnancy, well-woman care can be initiated. The relevant components include screening for obesity, lipid screening, and diabetes.[1] The goal of this screening is to identify disease among these women at high risk due to their prior pregnancy complications, excessive gestational weight gain, or obesity. Optimizing their health at this critical time can help in primary or secondary prevention.

SUMMARY

Obesity and excessive gestational weight gain are associated with adverse perinatal outcomes.[3] Excessive gestational weight gain often translates into postpartum weight retention and obesity, leading to lifelong impacts on maternal and child health.[5] Exercise and nutrition play a key role in reducing gestational weight gain, particularly in pregnancy, during which women are inherently motivated to make lifestyle modifications.[10] Obstetric providers should use the opportunity provided by pregnancy to inform women of their health risks and implement appropriate primary and second prevention strategies for women at risk of chronic disease. This is an initiative that should be undertaken by all health care providers caring for women of reproductive-age.[2]

REFERENCES

1. Initiative WPSI. Recommendations for well-woman care: a well-woman chart. Washington, DC: ACOG Foundation; 2018.
2. Smith GN, Saade G. SMFM white paper: pregnancy as a window to future health. SMFM Health Policy Committee. Available at: https://www.smfm.org/publications/141-smfm-white-paper-pregnancy-as-a-window-to-future-health. Accessed May 26, 2019.
3. Dolin CD, Kominiarek MA. Pregnancy in women with obesity. Obstet Gynecol Clin North Am 2018;45(2):217–32.
4. McDowoll M, Cain MA, Brumley J. Excessive gestational weight gain. J Midwifery Womens Health 2018. https://doi.org/10.1111/jmwh.12927.
5. Gilmore LA, Klempel-Donchenko M, Redman LM. Pregnancy as a window to future health: excessive gestational weight gain and obesity. Semin Perinatol 2015;39(4):296–303.
6. Yaniv-Salem S, Shoham-Vardi I, Kessous R, et al. Obesity in pregnancy: what's next? Long-term cardiovascular morbidity in a follow-up period of more than a decade. J Matern Fetal Neonatal Med 2016;29(4):619–23.
7. Louis JM, Bryant A, Ramos D, et al. Interpregnancy care. Am J Obstet Gynecol 2019;220(1):B2–18.
8. Amorim Adegboye AR, Linne YM. Diet or exercise, or both, for weight reduction in women after childbirth. Cochrane Database Syst Rev 2013;(7):CD005627.
9. Marchi J, Berg M, Dencker A, et al. Risks associated with obesity in pregnancy, for the mother and baby: a systematic review of reviews. Obes Rev 2015;16(8):621–38.
10. Farpour-Lambert NJ, Ells LJ, Martinez de Tejada B, et al. Obesity and weight gain in pregnancy and postpartum: an evidence review of lifestyle interventions to inform maternal and child health policies. Front Endocrinol (Lausanne) 2018;9:546.
11. Peaceman AM, Clifton RG, Phelan S, et al. Lifestyle interventions limit gestational weight gain in women with overweight or obesity: LIFE-moms prospective meta-analysis. Obesity 2018;26(9):1396–404.
12. Perales M, Artal R, Lucia A. Exercise during pregnancy. JAMA 2017;317(11):1113–4.
13. Nascimento SL, Surita FG, Cecatti JG. Physical exercise during pregnancy: a systematic review. Curr Opin Obstet Gynecol 2012;24(6):387–94.
14. Nnam NM. Improving maternal nutrition for better pregnancy outcomes. Proc Nutr Soc 2015;74(4):454–9.
15. Yang Z, Huffman SL. Nutrition in pregnancy and early childhood and associations with obesity in developing countries. Matern Child Nutr 2013;9(Suppl 1):105–19.

Menstrual Health as a Part of Preventive Health Care

Kristen A. Matteson, MD, MPH[a],*, Kate M. Zaluski, MD[b]

KEYWORDS

- Menstrual health • Normal uterine bleeding • Abnormal uterine bleeding
- Endometriosis • Premenstrual syndrome

KEY POINTS

- Assessment of menstrual health is a key component of well-woman care. Some women, unprompted, may not disclose symptoms related to their menstrual cycle that may represent an underlying health problem.
- A normal menstrual cycle is the coordinated synchronous bleeding and cessation of bleeding of a normal endometrium and uterus orchestrated by estrogen and progesterone influence and their abrupt withdrawal.
- Asking questions about the frequency, duration, regularity, and volume of uterine bleeding will help identify a woman who is experiencing abnormal uterine bleeding.
- The PALM-COEIN system can be used to develop a differential diagnosis for the symptom of abnormal uterine bleeding.
- Conditions, other than abnormal uterine bleeding, that could be diagnosed in the process of a comprehensive menstrual health evaluation include endometriosis, dysmenorrhea, and premenstrual syndrome.

INTRODUCTION

The American College of Obstetricians and Gynecologists (ACOG) recommends that, for adolescents, an evaluation of the menstrual cycle should be included as a vital sign because it can improve the early identification of potential health problems.[1] Using this same rationale, evaluation of the menstrual cycles and symptoms associated with it, referred to within this article as menstrual health, are essential components of well-woman care for adult women.[2] Menstrual health assessment facilitates identification of a pathologic condition (eg, abnormal uterine bleeding [AUB], endometriosis), offers

[a] Division of Research, Department of Obstetrics and Gynecology, Women and Infants Hospital, Warren Alpert Medical School of Brown University, 101 Dudley Street, Providence, RI 02905, USA; [b] Division of Emergency Obstetrics and Gynecology, Department of Obstetrics and Gynecology, Women and Infants Hospital, Warren Alpert Medical School of Brown University, 101 Dudley Street, Providence, RI 02905, USA
* Corresponding author.
E-mail address: KMatteson@wihri.org

Obstet Gynecol Clin N Am 46 (2019) 441–453
https://doi.org/10.1016/j.ogc.2019.04.004
0889-8545/19/© 2019 Elsevier Inc. All rights reserved.

obgyn.theclinics.com

the opportunity to educate women on what menstrual symptoms may be normal or abnormal, and provides the opportunity to initiate treatment of women who are suffering because of problems with their menstrual bleeding or associated symptoms. In the scientific vision statement for the Gynecologic Health and Disease Research branch of the National Institute of Child Health and Human Development, Tingen and colleagues[3] stated that lack of education and stigma result in barriers to care for gynecologic health disorders, and that women often suffer in silence because they have a difficult time expressing their symptoms to their physicians or they think their symptoms are an inevitable outcome of menstruation.

Because some women, unprompted, may not disclose symptoms related to their menstrual cycle that could represent an underlying problem, including heavy menstrual bleeding, pain, or mood disorders, either because of embarrassment or because they think their suffering is normal, health care providers need to be familiar with menstrual health disorders and take a thorough history to assist women in discussing their menstrual health experiences. This article describes menstrual health, first in terms of the physiologic process of menstruation and the normal parameters of menstrual bleeding. Next, it covers the diagnosis and evaluation of AUB and a brief description of other nonbleeding menstrual health disorders, including dysmenorrhea, endometriosis, and premenstrual syndrome (PMS).

Impact of Menstrual Health Problems on Women

In the United States, each year, more than 4.5 million reproductive-aged women experience at least one gynecologic health problem, and the most common problems are related to menstrual health, which encompasses a wide range of issues, including AUB, dysmenorrhea, endometriosis, and PMS.[4] AUB affects up to 1.5 million women annually. In the United States, it is associated with $1 billion annually in direct costs and $12 to $36 billion in indirect costs if lost work wages and productivity are included.[5–7] Dysmenorrhea, painful menstruation, occurs in 50% to 90% of women and is the most common reason adolescents are repeatedly absent from school.[8] The most common cause of secondary dysmenorrhea, endometriosis, affects 6% to 10% of reproductive-age women and costs $49 billion annually in terms of diagnosis and treatment.[9,10] However, because some women may have endometriosis without symptoms, it is difficult to determine the exact prevalence and costs of this condition. Similarly, PMS is extremely common and can have a significant impact on a woman's well-being. A hallmark of each of these menstrual health conditions is that the symptoms associated with them, from heavy bleeding, to pain, to fatigue and mood changes, have a significant impact on a woman's physical, social, and emotional quality of life. Promptly identifying and treating these disorders by incorporating their assessment into routine well-woman care has the potential to positively affect the lives of a substantial number of women.

NORMAL MENSTRUAL BLEEDING AND THE HYPOTHALAMUS-PITUITARY-OVARY-ENDOMETRIUM AXIS

A normal menstrual cycle is the coordinated synchronous bleeding and cessation of bleeding of a normal endometrium and uterus orchestrated by estrogen and progesterone influence and their abrupt withdrawal. Normal cycles depend on the event of ovulation, which occurs via a coordinated cascade of hormonal signals with positive and negative feedback loops in the hypothalamus-pituitary-ovary-endometrium axis.

The first part of the menstrual cycle, the follicular phase, starts with the onset of menses and varies in length between women. Pulsatile release of gonadotropin-releasing hormone from the hypothalamus causes the anterior pituitary to secrete follicle-stimulating hormone (FSH). This FSH acts on the ovary to recruit a cohort of antral follicles. These antral follicles and their supporting stromal cells secrete estrogen; the follicles most successful at producing estrogen become the (usually single) dominant follicle, which will eventually ovulate. The estrogen released from the dominant follicle both positively feeds back to the anterior pituitary to release a surge of luteinizing hormone (LH) and stimulates the growth of the endometrium.

The latter portion of the menstrual cycle is the luteal phase, which is uniformly 13 to 15 days in length in all women. The luteal phase starts with the LH surge, which then stimulates ovulation. After the ovum is released, progesterone is produced by the remains of the dominant follicle, which is now called the corpus luteum. This progesterone causes decidualization of the endometrial lining of the uterus. If the released oocyte is not fertilized, the corpus luteum ceases to provide progesterone and the withdrawal of both estrogen and progesterone leads to the decidualized endometrium shedding in an orderly fashion, causing menstruation.

Immediately after menses, during the follicular phase, the endometrium reepithelializes and the hormonally responsive functionalis layer grows (approximately 3–4 mm) under the influence of estrogen secreted from the ovaries. The progesterone released in response to ovulation stops the rapid growth of endometrium and initiates a precise sequence of secretory changes to the glands (decidualization). The glands become more tortuous, the stroma more edematous, and the spiral arteries more coiled, all in preparation for a possible implantation.

In the absence of implantation, ovarian estrogen and progesterone levels decrease, which by multiple molecular pathways (prostaglandin, cytokine, metalloproteinase activity, vascular endothelial growth factor expression) leads to endometrial sloughing. After the menstrual onset, the process of hemostasis is complex and multifactorial. Vasoconstriction of the spiral arteries is stimulated by prostaglandins and endothelins found in the endometrium. Coagulation is aided by local tissue factors, which promote clotting, as well as platelet plugs. The basalis layer quickly regenerates from the residual portions of glands until the entire uterine cavity is covered, after which stem cells from the basalis layer recreate the stromal portion of the endometrium.

EVALUATION OF MENSTRUAL HEALTH (BLEEDING AND ASSOCIATED SYMPTOMS)

Normal uterine bleeding is the result of the physiologic process of the menstrual cycle (previously outlined) in women before menopause, which is defined as the final menstrual period resulting from the physiologic permanent decline in gonadal hormone levels confirmed by 12 months of amenorrhea in women with a uterus.[11,12] Postmenopausal bleeding, defined as bleeding from female genital organs 12 or more months after the final menstrual period, affects up to 10% of women. Although it can be caused by nonmalignant etiologic factors, postmenopausal bleeding can be caused by endometrial cancer and hyperplasia, and always warrants evaluation (see later discussion of special considerations).[13,14]

Parameters of Typical Menstrual Bleeding in Reproductive Aged Women: Frequency, Regularity, Duration, and Volume

To address problems with inconsistent and poorly defined terminologies, the Menstrual Disorders Committee (MDC) of the International Federation of Gynecologists and Obstetricians (FIGO) published recommendations for standardized terminologies related to menstrual bleeding and AUB.[15–17] For use in both clinical and research settings, the FIGO MDC recommends describing bleeding symptoms in terms of 4 menstrual dimensions: frequency, regularity, duration, and volume (**Table 1**).[17]

These definitions of normal menstrual bleeding were adopted by ACOG through the reVITALize Gynecology Data Definitions Initiative, a process started in 2013 to standardize the definitions of common reproductive health terminologies for use in documentation, research, coding, and databases.[11,12] The terminologies and definitions developed as part of this process are outlined in **Table 2**. Understanding the normal range of these dimensions is a critical first step in diagnosing and treating menstrual health disorders.

These definitions may continue to evolve as more data, potentially from more diverse populations, become available to contribute to the definition of population norms for menstrual bleeding. The definition of 1 parameter of bleeding, volume, has evolved considerably over the past decade to move away from strictly defining it objectively as greater than 80 mL of menstrual blood loss per cycle, which was not relevant to clinical care or feasible to measure in clinical practice, to defining it in a more patient-centered way that focuses on the impact of the bleeding on the woman's quality of life (see **Tables 1** and **2**).

Asking questions to categorize a woman's bleeding relative to these 4 dimensions will facilitate consistent description of bleeding patterns between clinical providers and the ability to identify a woman who is experiencing AUB. However, AUB is not the only menstrual health disorder and, as such, an evaluation of these 4 dimensions alone is too superficial to determine whether or not a woman is experiencing other associated symptoms related to her menses and whether or not her bleeding is having a negative impact on her quality of life. Multiple validated questionnaires have been developed to evaluate both menstrual bleeding and related menstrual symptoms with regard to quality of life.[18,19] Additionally, asking questions about associated symptoms, such as pain and mood changes, as part of a comprehensive evaluation of menstrual health may facilitate the diagnosis of endometriosis, dysmenorrhea, PMS, or major premenstrual dysphoric disorder (PMDD). See later discussion of these disorders and their assessment in the context of preventive health.

Table 1 The International Federation of Gynecologists and Obstetricians Menstrual Disorders Committee uterine bleeding classification system (system 1)		
Frequency	Frequent	Less than every 24 d
	Normal	Every 24–38 d
	Infrequent	Every 38 d
	Absent	No periods or bleeding: amenorrhea
Regularity	Regular	Variation (shortest to longest) ≤9 d
	Irregular	Variation (shortest to longest) >10
Duration	Prolonged	>8 d
	Normal	≤8 d
Volume	Heavy	Determined by the patient
	Normal	Heavy menstrual bleeding defined as bleeding sufficient to cause
	Light	interference with quality of life

The FIGO symptom classification system was revised in 2018. This table represents these changes to the system.

Adapted from Munro MG, Critchley HOD, Fraser IS, et al. The two FIGO systems for normal and abnormal uterine bleeding symptoms and classification of causes of abnormal uterine bleeding in the reproductive years: 2018 revisions. Int J Gynaecol Obstet 2018;143(3):393–408; with permission.

Table 2 The American College of Obstetricians and Gynecologists reVITALize data definitions gynecology related to bleeding	
Normal uterine bleeding	Cyclic bleeding that occurs from the uterine corpus between menarche and menopause The bleeding generally lasts up to 8 d and occurs every 24–38 d The cycle should occur at regular predictable intervals and the difference between the longest and shortest cycle over a 1-year period should be no more than 20 d[a] Normal volume may be defined quantitatively as up to 80 mL per cycle and/or qualitatively as volume that does not excessively interfere with a woman's physical, social, emotional, and/or material quality of life
AUB	Bleeding from the uterus that differs in frequency, regularity, duration, or volume from normal uterine bleeding, in the absence of pregnancy AUB as a symptom should be further classified etiologically as follows: PALM-COEIN: polyp, adenomyosis, leiomyoma, malignancy and hyperplasia, coagulopathy, ovulatory dysfunction, endometrial, iatrogenic, and not otherwise classified
Heavy menstrual bleeding (formerly menorrhagia)	A type of AUB characterized by excessive cyclic blood loss, which differs from normal uterine bleeding and interferes with a woman's physical, social, emotional, and/or material quality of life
Irregular and heavy uterine bleeding (formerly menometrorrhagia)	A type of AUB that represents the symptom of excessive uterine blood loss (in terms of volume or duration) which occurs unpredictably and interferes with a woman's physical, social, emotional, and/or material quality of life
Intermenstrual bleeding	A type of AUB characterized by bleeding episodes between regular episodes of cyclic uterine bleeding
Postmenopausal bleeding	Bleeding from female genital organs $\geq$12 mo after the final menstrual period

[a] The 20-day difference was based on the 2011 FIGO MDC work and on a general population of women, including women with very short (<18 day) and very long (>43 day) cycles. When these women are excluded, variation is age-dependent and is typically 7 to 9 days. The FIGO MDC has changed their definition of regularity to exclude women with very short and very long cycles.

Data from American College of Obstetricians and Gynecologists (ACOG). reVITALize Gynecology Data Definitions (Version 1.0). Available at: https://www.acog.org/-/media/Departments/Patient-Safety-and-Quality-Improvement/reVITALize-Gynecology-Definitons-V1.pdf?dmc=1&ts=2019010 7T1517060047. Accessed January 4, 2019.

Developing a Differential Diagnosis for Abnormal Uterine Bleeding

If there is suspicion of a menstrual health disorder, a focused physical examination followed by laboratory testing and imaging, as indicated, should be conducted to narrow down the differential diagnosis and determine the most likely cause to assist in selecting the appropriate management strategy. Assessment for pregnancy is often the first step in evaluation because the workup of bleeding in pregnancy (beyond the scope of this article) would be very different from workup for bleeding in a nonpregnant reproductive-age woman. In addition to ruling out pregnancy, history and physical examination can be helpful to differentiate uterine bleeding from vaginal, cervical, or urinary sources.

Once pregnancy and other sources of bleeding in the genital tract have been eliminated, a workup should be undertaken to determine the cause of the AUB, which is a symptom and not a diagnosis in and of itself. In addition to the symptom description system (see **Table 1**), the FIGO MDC developed a separate system to describe the etiologic factors that are associated with AUB, including polyps, adenomyosis, leiomyomas, malignancy (and hyperplasia), coagulopathy, ovulatory dysfunction, endometrial dysfunction, iatrogenic, and not otherwise classified (PALM-COEIN).[15–17] The PALM-COEIN system (see **Table 3**) is valuable in both clinical practice and research settings for standardizing language related to the differential diagnosis of AUB, selecting testing to narrow down the differential diagnosis, and in counseling related to AUB management strategies. The PALM portion of the acronym refers to the structural causes within the uterus that may lead to AUB, whereas the COFIN portion refers to nonstructural pathologic conditions leading to AUB (**Table 3**).[15–17]

Structural Causes of Abnormal Uterine Bleeding

Polyps

Endometrial polyps are localized overgrowths of endometrial glands and stroma around a vascular core. Most uterine polyps are benign but may rarely contain malignancy. Patients with polyps may report intermenstrual or heavy menstrual bleeding. It is challenging to estimate how common endometrial polyps are because many are asymptomatic. A review of the literature shows a wide range of prevalence estimates, from 7.8% to 34.9%, which seem to increase with increasing age.[20] Additional risk factors include tamoxifen use and obesity, which affects long-term health. (See Drs Elizabeth A. Hoover and Judette M. Louis's article, "Optimizing Health: Weight, Exercise, and Nutrition in Pregnancy and Beyond," in this issue.) The size and number of polyps do not necessarily correlate with degree of symptoms. Polyps may regress or be shed with menstrual bleeding. Because most polyps are intracavitary, there will not often be findings on physical examination unless the polyp is prolapsing through the cervix.

Adenomyosis

Adenomyosis occurs when endometrial glands are present within the myometrium, which also may be hypertrophic. It can be associated with AUB but also may be present in women who are asymptomatic. Symptomatic patients with adenomyosis may note excessively heavy and painful menses. Prevalence is very difficult to estimate because diagnosis can only be made definitively on pathologic assessment posthysterectomy. Several findings on ultrasound indicate adenomyosis; the FIGO MDC is working on a consensus system to classify imaging findings diagnostic for

Table 3
The International Federation of Gynecologists and Obstetricians PALM-COEIN system of classifying the causes of abnormal uterine bleeding (system 2)

PALM: Structural Causes		COEIN: Nonstructural Causes	
Polyp	AUB-P	Coagulopathy	AUB-C
Adenomyosis	AUB-A	Ovulatory dysfunction	AUB-O
Leiomyoma	AUB-L	Endometrial	AUB-E
Malignancy and hyperplasia	AUB-M	Iatrogenic	AUB-I
—	—	Not otherwise classified	AUB-N

Adapted from Munro MG, Critchley HO, Broder MS, et al. FIGO classification system (PALM-COEIN) for causes of abnormal uterine bleeding in nongravid women of reproductive age. Int J Gynaecol Obstet 2011;113(1):3–13; with permission.

adenomyosis.[17] An enlarged and globular uterus on physical examination, which may be tender to palpation, suggests the diagnosis of adenomyosis.

Leiomyomas

Leiomyomas, also known as uterine fibroids, are benign monoclonal tumors of smooth muscle cells within the myometrium. One study that used ultrasound to screen women for leiomyoma independent of clinical symptoms found a cumulative incidence by age 49 years of 70% for white women and 80% for black women.[21] Symptomatic leiomyoma may result in heavy menstrual bleeding, bulk symptoms, infertility, or obstetric complications. Not all patients will have symptoms, which depend on the number, size, and location of leiomyoma. Findings may include an enlarged or irregular uterus on bimanual examination.

Malignancy and hyperplasia

Endometrial cancer and hyperplasia of the endometrium, though less common causes of AUB in premenopausal women, must be ruled out in women with risk factors. Risk factors for endometrial hyperplasia and cancer include long-standing unopposed estrogen exposure (eg, in the case of polycystic ovarian syndrome [PCOS] and obesity), women for whom treatment of heavy menstrual bleeding has been unsuccessful, and women taking tamoxifen.[22,23] In postmenopausal women with uterine bleeding, endometrial cancer and hyperplasia are much more common. Approximately 9% of women with postmenopausal bleeding will be diagnosed with endometrial cancer.[13] See later discussion of special considerations for endometrial biopsy evaluation for malignancy and hyperplasia.

Nonstructural Causes of Abnormal Uterine Bleeding

Coagulopathy

AUB may be caused by coagulopathy, which refers to systemic disorders of hemostasis. Hemostasis disorders may be due to bleeding diathesis (von Willebrand disease, immune thrombocytopenia, inherited or acquired platelet function defect) or systemic disease (liver or kidney disease). The most common inherited bleeding disorder, von Willebrand disease, has been found in 13% of women with heavy menstrual bleeding.[24] Bleeding patterns may be variable but most commonly would present as heavy or prolonged menstrual bleeding, usually since menarche in the case of inherited bleeding disorders. Obtaining a focused medical history and clinical screening for disorders of hemostasis (**Box 1**) in women with heavy menstrual bleeding will assist in determining which patients should have diagnostic laboratory testing.[25] Patients with a positive screen should have further laboratory evaluation and consideration of a consultation with a hematologist.

Ovulatory dysfunction

Ovulatory dysfunction encompasses a wide range of etiologic factors, including hypothalamic dysfunction, pituitary or thyroid disorders, and PCOS, and therefore has a wide range of menstrual bleeding presentations, including amenorrhea. Typically, ovulatory dysfunction results in irregular, unpredictable episodes of uterine bleeding of varying duration and varying volume. A detailed clinical history related to bleeding pattern can facilitate the diagnosis of AUB–ovulatory dysfunction. Taking a detailed history medical history (other associated symptoms; ie, hirsutism, acne, headaches, vision changes, fatigue) can help facilitate the selection of appropriate laboratory and/or imaging to narrow down the differential diagnosis.[17]

> **Box 1**
> **Medical history and initial clinical screening for disorders of hemostasis in women with heavy menstrual bleeding**
>
> *Recommend laboratory evaluation for disorders of hemostasis in women with heavy menstrual bleeding since menarche*
>
> Plus 1 of the following symptoms
>   Postpartum hemorrhage
>   Surgical-related bleeding
>   Bleeding associated with dental work
>
> Or 2 or more of the following symptoms
>   Bruising 1 to 2 times per month
>   Epistaxis 1 to 2 times per month
>   Frequent gum bleeding
>   Family history of bleeding symptoms
>
> *Adapted from* Kouides PA, Conard J, Peyvandi F, et al. Hemostasis and menstruation: appropriate investigation for underlying disorders of hemostasis in women with excessive menstrual bleeding. Fertility and Sterility 2005;84(5):1345–51.

Endometrial dysfunction

Endometrial dysfunction occurs when there is compromised hemostasis within the endometrium itself, which may present as heavy or prolonged menstrual bleeding. Processes affected in endometrial dysfunction include endometrial deficits in vasoconstriction, accelerated lysis of endometrial clot, and other local molecular mechanisms responsible for hemostasis. Unfortunately, there are no clinically available tests to confirm a diagnosis of endometrial dysfunction. Therefore, endometrial dysfunction is often a diagnosis of exclusion in a patient with historically regular and predictable cycles, characteristic of ovulatory cycles, but for whom a workup fails to reveal another cause.

Iatrogenic

Iatrogenic causes of AUB are due to medications or medical interventions. The most common cause of AUB–iatrogenic is from the use of steroid hormone (estrogen and/or progestin) medications. In these cases, bleeding is usually characterized as unscheduled or breakthrough bleeding. Other medical therapies that can cause AUB–iatrogenic include those that interfere with dopamine metabolism and those associated with anticoagulant medication or chemotherapy.[17]

Not otherwise classified

A final category of AUB, not otherwise classified, is reserved for etiologic factors that are not well understood but may contribute to the symptom of AUB. Chronic endometritis, arteriovenous malformations, cesarean section niche, and myometrial hypertrophy are examples of entities that may be associated with AUB but have not been well-studied or defined.

ARRIVING AT A DIAGNOSIS: CONSIDERATIONS FOR PHYSICAL EXAMINATION, LABORATORY TESTING, AND IMAGING
Physical Examination

A physical examination should be offered to all women with AUB or other related menstrual symptoms. Although there is a lack of data to support the effectiveness of a routine pelvic examination as a screening tool for an asymptomatic patient at a well-woman visit, in the case of suspected AUB or endometriosis, a pelvic examination should be recommended to the patient.[26]

Laboratory Testing

The selection of laboratory tests should be based on the complex of symptoms the woman reports. A complete blood count is recommended for all women presenting with heavy menstrual bleeding and a pregnancy test for all women at risk for pregnancy. Additional testing may include a thyroid-stimulating hormone level, chlamydia and gonorrhea testing, and targeted screening for bleeding disorders if indicated based on responses to screening.[22] Based on the guidelines published by the ACOG, endometrial tissue sampling should be considered a first-line test in women with AUB age 45 years and older and women under the age of 45 years with risk factors (previously described) to evaluate for endometrial hyperplasia and cancer.[22] It should be mentioned that recommendations for testing are not the same across all clinical care environments; different guidelines for laboratory testing and endometrial sampling are published in the United Kingdom.[23]

Imaging

Although uterine imaging, by transvaginal ultrasound or hysteroscopy, can assist with the diagnosis of structural abnormalities, it does not need to be performed at initial evaluation for AUB.[22,23] In cases in which pelvic examination reveals structural abnormalities, there is clinical suspicion of structural abnormality, or a patient has not responded as expected to treatment, uterine imaging can be performed. Choice of imaging (transvaginal ultrasound vs hysteroscopy) should be based on a suspected pathologic condition.

Special Considerations: Postmenopausal Women

Methods for endometrial evaluation among women with postmenopausal bleeding include transvaginal ultrasound, endometrial tissue sampling, and hysteroscopy combined with endometrial sampling.[27] Test selection is based on the availability of the testing modalities, patient factors, and patient and clinician preferences.[14] Transvaginal ultrasonography can be used as a first-line test in women with postmenopausal bleeding because an endometrial echo thickness less than or equal to 4 mm has a 99% negative predictive value for endometrial cancer. Patients with endometrial thickness greater than 4 mm or with recurrent bleeding should have endometrial sampling.[27] Endometrial sampling is also an acceptable first-line method of evaluation. Persistent or recurrent bleeding requires additional evaluation (hysteroscopy with endometrial sampling), even in women with benign blind endometrial sampling.[14,27]

CONSIDERATIONS FOR TREATMENT OF ABNORMAL UTERINE BLEEDING IN REPRODUCTIVE AGED WOMEN

Both surgical and medical options are available to treat AUB. A side benefit of access to contraceptive choices is the treatment of menstrual irregularities. (See Nichole Tyson's article, "Reproductive Health: Options, Strategies, and Empowerment of Women," in this issue.) When offering women treatment of their symptoms of heavy or irregular menstrual bleeding, the cause (PALM-COEIN) needs to be considered because appropriate treatment options and the effectiveness of the treatment options vary by the cause (PALM-COEIN) of the AUB. Determining the underlying etiologic factors of AUB is not always simple. For example, in the process of evaluating a woman for heavy menstrual bleeding, uterine leiomyomas are commonly identified by ultrasound. However, it is impossible to determine if these leiomyomas are the actual cause of the bleeding and not an incidental finding, especially if the leiomyomas are not submucosal. Treatment effectiveness is not the only consideration when selecting treatment options for AUB. Other considerations when choosing treatments to decrease a woman's menstrual bleeding and improve her quality of life are contraindications to the individual treatment options, comorbid conditions, availability, cost, other treatments previously tried, desire (or lack of desire) for contraception, other associated conditions (eg, endometriosis, dysmenorrhea, PMS, or PMDD). Taking a detailed history to help elucidate the cause of the AUB and evaluating patient values, preferences, and expectations related to treatment can provide a patient-centered approach to initial care of a woman experiencing AUB. A full discussion of treatment options for the symptom of AUB is outside of the scope of this article.

BEYOND THE BLEEDING: OTHER MENSTRUAL HEALTH SYMPTOMS

Assessment of menstrual health goes beyond assessing the timing, frequency, duration, and volume of bleeding, and the impact of bleeding on quality of life, and includes assessment of other symptoms, such as pain and mood changes and the woman's family planning needs. Conditions with symptoms related to menstrual bleeding include endometriosis, dysmenorrhea, PMS, and PMDD. Identifying these conditions as part of the well-woman evaluation provides the opportunity for patient education, treatment, and appropriate patient follow-up.

Dysmenorrhea

Dysmenorrhea can be primary (in the absence of pelvic disease) or secondary (due to a coexisting medical problem or pelvic disease), with the most common cause of secondary dysmenorrhea being endometriosis. Many women experience a delay in evaluation and diagnosis and cite perceived lack of physician interest in pain symptoms as a barrier to care-seeking.[28] All women should be asked questions about pain during menses to facilitate the diagnosis and conversations about treatment of dysmenorrhea, and taking a detailed medical and menstrual history can assist with determining if the woman has primary or secondary dysmenorrhea.

Endometriosis

Endometriosis is a chronic condition and can have a significant impact on physical, social, and emotional quality of life. Presentation of symptoms to diagnosis of endometriosis, on average, takes 7 to 8 years, which suggests that health care professionals may not be considering endometriosis on the differential diagnosis and may not be asking the right questions to facilitate the diagnosis.[9] Endometriosis should be suspected in adolescents and women with chronic pelvic pain, dysmenorrhea affecting daily activities and quality of life, dyspareunia, period-related gastrointestinal symptoms (specifically painful bowel movements), period-related or cyclical urinary symptoms, or infertility.[29] Asking questions about these symptoms can ensure they are being addressed and endometriosis is being considered as an etiologic factor. Delay in diagnosis and treatment of endometriosis has an adverse impact on quality of life.

Premenstrual Syndrome and Premenstrual Dysphoric Disorder

PMS is characterized by the presence of physical symptoms (eg, joint pain, breast tenderness or swelling, abdominal bloating, headaches, skin disorders, weight gain) or affective symptoms (eg, depression, fatigue, mood swings, irritability, anxiety, confusion, hopelessness) that are present during the luteal phase of the menstrual cycle and disappear by the end of menstruation, and range from mild to severe.[30] A severe form of PMS, PMDD is characterized by the presence of at least 5 affective symptoms that cause functional impairment in the final week before the onset of menses that improve within a few days after the onset of menses, and resolve in the week postmenses; however, specific American Psychiatric Association criteria (*Diagnostic and Statistical Manual of Mental Disorders*, 5th edition) need to be met for the diagnosis of PMDD.[30,31] To enable the prompt and proper diagnosis of PMS and PMDD, women should be asked questions about whether or not they experience these hallmark symptoms, specifically mood-related symptoms, before their menstrual period and, if present, what impact these symptoms have on their work, social, and family life.

SUMMARY

Women spend nearly half of their lives experiencing menstrual bleeding. Abnormalities in the volume or pattern of menstrual bleeding and symptoms associated with menstrual bleeding, such as pain or anxiety, can have a significant impact on a woman's quality of life. Assessment of menstrual health can provide an opportunity to educate women on what is normal, and what is not, and identification of a patient who is suffering from a variety of health problems ranging from endometriosis to AUB to PMDD. Postmenopausal women should be educated that vaginal bleeding can be a symptom of endometrial cancer and that they should seek medical attention for this symptom. Comprehensive menstrual health assessment should be incorporated as an essential component of well-woman care.

REFERENCES

1. ACOG Committee Opinion No. 651: menstruation in girls and adolescents: using the menstrual cycle as a vital sign. Obstet Gynecol 2015;126(6):e143–6.
2. ACOG annual well-woman exam infographic. Available at: https://www.acog.org/Patients/FAQs/Annual-Well-Woman-Exam-Infographic. Accessed January 4, 2019.
3. Tingen CM, Mazloomdoost D, Halvorson L. Gynecologic health and disease research at the Eunice Kennedy Shriver National Institute of Child Health and Human Development, A scientific vision. Obstet Gynecol 2018;132:987–98.
4. Kjerulff KH, Erickson BA, Langenberg PW. Chronic gynecological conditions reported by US women: findings from the National Health Interview Survey, 1984 to 1992. Am J Public Health 1996;86(2):195–9.
5. Matteson KA, Raker CA, Clark MA, et al. Abnormal uterine bleeding, health status, and usual source of medical care: analyses using the medical expenditures panel survey. J Womens Health 2013;22(11):959–65.
6. Cote I, Jacobs P, Cumming D. Work loss associated with increased menstrual loss in the United States. Obstet Gynecol 2002;100(4):683–7.
7. Cote I, Jacobs P, Cumming DC. Use of health services associated with increased menstrual loss in the United States. Am J Obstet Gynecol 2003;188(2):343–8.
8. Dysmenorrhea and endometriosis in the adolescent. Committee Opinion Number 760. American College of Obstetricians and Gynecologists. Obstet Gynecol 2018;132:e249–58.
9. Falcone T, Flyckt R. Clinical management of endometriosis. Obstet Gynecol 2018; 13:557–71.
10. Simoens S, Dunselman G, Dirksen C, et al. The burden of endometriosis: costs and quality of life of women with endometriosis and treated in referral centres. Humanit Rep 2012;27:1292–9.

11. Sharp HT, Johnson JV, Lemieux LA, et al. Executive summary of the reVITALize initiative: standardizing gynecologic data definitions. Obstet Gynecol 2017; 129(4):603–7.

12. ACOG reVITALize Gynecology data definitions website. Available at: https://www. acog.org/-/media/Departments/Patient-Safety-and-Quality-Improvement/reVITA Lize-Gynecology-Definitons-V1.pdf?dmc=1&ts=20190107T1517060047. Accessed January 4, 2019.

13. Clarke MA, Long BJ, Del Mar Morillo A, et al. Association of endometrial cancer risk with postmenopausal bleeding in women: a systematic review and meta-analysis. JAMA Intern Med 2018;178(9):1210–22.

14. Matteson KA, Robison K, Jacoby VL. Opportunities for early detection of endometrial cancer in women with postmenopausal bleeding. JAMA Intern Med 2018;178(9):1222–3.

15. Munro M, Critchley H, Broder M, et al. FIGO classification system (PALM-COEIN) for causes of abnormal uterine bleeding in nongravid women of reproductive age. Int J Gynecol Obstet 2011;113(1):3–13.

16. Munro MG, Critchley HO, Fraser IS, FIGO Menstrual Disorders Working Group. The FIGO classification of causes of abnormal uterine bleeding in the reproductive years. Fertil Steril 2011;95(7):2204–8.

17. Munro MG, Critchley HOD, Fraser IS, et al. The two FIGO systems for normal and abnormal uterine bleeding symptoms and classification of causes of abnormal uterine bleeding in the reproductive years: 2018 revisions. Int J Gynecol Obstet 2018;143(3):393–408.

18. Matteson KA, Boardman LA, Munro MG, et al. Abnormal uterine bleeding: a review of patient-based outcome measures. Fertil Steril 2009;92(1):205–16.

19. Matteson KA, Scott DM, Raker CA, et al. The menstrual bleeding questionnaire: development and validation of a comprehensive patient-reported outcome instrument for heavy menstrual bleeding. BJOG 2015;122(5):681–9.

20. Salim S, Won H, Nesbitt-Hawes E, et al. Diagnosis and management of endometrial polyps: a critical review of the literature. J Minim Invasive Gynecol 2011; 18(5):569–81.

21. Baird DD, Dunson DB, Hill MC, et al. High cumulative incidence of uterine leiomyoma in black and white women: Ultrasound evidence. Am J Obstet Gynecol 2003;188(1):100–7.

22. Committee on Practice Bulletins—Gynecology. Practice bulletin no. 128: diagnosis of abnormal uterine bleeding in reproductive-aged women. Obstet Gynecol 2012;120(1):197–206.

23. National Institute for Health and Care Excellence. Heavy menstrual bleeding: assessment and management (NICE Guideline No. 88). 2018. Available at: https://www.nice.org.uk/guidance/ng88.

24. Kadir RA, Economides DL, Sabin CA, et al. Frequency of inherited bleeding disorders in women with menorrhagia. Lancet 1998;351(9101):485–9.

25. Kouides PA, Conard J, Peyvandi F, et al. Hemostasis and menstruation: appropriate investigation for underlying disorders of hemostasis in women with excessive menstrual bleeding. Fertil Steril 2005;84(5):1345–51.

26. ACOG Committee Opinion No. 754: the utility of and indications for routine pelvic examination. Obstet Gynecol 2018;132(4):e174–80.

27. ACOG Committee Opinion No. 734: the role of transvaginal ultrasonography in evaluating the endometrium of women with postmenopausal bleeding. Obstet Gynecol 2018;131(5):e124–9.

28. Mann J, Shuster J, Moawad N. Attributes and barriers to care of pelvic pain in university women. J Minim Invasive Gynecol 2013;20:811–8.
29. National Institute for Health and Care Excellence. Endometriosis: diagnosis and management (NICE Guideline No. 73). 2017. Available at: https://www.nice.org.uk/guidance/ng73.
30. Yonkers KA, Simoni MK. Premenstrual disorders. Am J Obstet Gynecol 2018;218(1):68–74.
31. American Psychiatric Association. Diagnostic and statistical manual of mental disorders. 5th edition. Washington, DC: American Psychiatric Association; 2013.

Environmental Exposures in Reproductive Health

Kelly McCue, MD[a], Nathaniel DeNicola, MD, MSHP[b],*

KEYWORDS

- Environmental health • Women's health • Reproductive health • Toxic exposures
- BPA • Air pollution • Pesticides

KEY POINTS

- Women's health providers play a vital role in protecting pregnancies from harmful environmental exposures.
- Pregnancy and the fetal period is perhaps the most critical time-window for human development, when any toxic exposure during can cause lasting damage to brain development and interfere with a child's ability to reach his or her full potential.
- Scientific consensus has identified several toxic chemical exposures that contribute to neurodevelopmental disorders such as attention deficit hyperactivity disorder and autism: organophosphate pesticides, polybrominated diphenyl ether (PBDE) flame retardants, combustion-related air pollutants, lead, mercury, and polychlorinated biphenyls (often used in carbonless copy paper).
- Reproductive care professionals do not need to be experts in environmental health science to provide useful information to patients and refer patients to appropriate specialists when a hazardous exposure is identified.

INTRODUCTION

Our genetic makeup and our environment interact to affect our health. The American College of Obstetricians and Gynecologists (ACOG) and the American Society on Reproductive Medicine have identified that robust scientific evidence has emerged over the past 25 years demonstrating that preconception and prenatal exposure to toxic environmental agents can have a profound and lasting effect on reproductive health across the life course.[1] Chemicals enter our environment worldwide as a result of our industrialized agricultural systems, through energy production, emissions, through production of consumer products, and waste disposal. Although chemicals

Disclosure: The authors have nothing to disclose.
[a] Obstetrics and Gynecology, The Permanente Medical Group, North Valley, 3rd Floor, 501 J Street, Sacramento, CA 95814, USA; [b] The George Washington University, 2511 I Street Northwest, Washington, DC 20037, USA
* Corresponding author.
E-mail address: ndenicola@gmail.com

are ubiquitous in our air, water, and our food, lower-income communities bear a disproportionate burden of exposure.[2]

Although we cannot change our genetics, we can change our environment, and there is growing consensus that we need to know how. Unlike with pharmaceuticals in the United States, the burden of proving safety has not been the responsibility of chemical manufacturers. The Frank R. Lautenberg Chemical Safety for the 21st Century Act amended the Toxic Substances Control Act (TSCA) in June of 2016, for the first time requiring the US Environmental Protection Agency (EPA) to evaluate existing chemicals using risk-based assessments.[3] The TSCA Inventory is composed of more than 85,000 chemicals,[4] of which 40,000 are active chemicals recognized as needing to be prioritized for evaluation.[5] However, even under the new law, the US EPA can still assess only a handful of chemicals a year.[6,7] The regulatory system for chemicals used in food and food packaging has similar deficits.[8]

ENVIRONMENTAL EXPOSURES AND WOMEN'S AND REPRODUCTIVE HEALTH

Before delving into types of environmental exposures, it is important to consider the vital role of women's health providers in protecting pregnancies from harm.[9] Because pregnancy and the fetal period is perhaps the most critical time-window for human development, toxic exposures during this time may lead to lasting damage to brain development and interfere with a child's ability to reach his or her full potential (Project TENDR [Targeting Environmental Neuro-Developmental Risk]). Every women's health care provider will encounter opportunities for counseling. Toxic chemicals are so numerous that every pregnant woman is likely exposed at some point in gestation to over 60 chemicals.[10,11]

Our environment, including exposure to toxicants and pollution, can affect future generations through epigenetics. Epigenetics includes the study of heritable phenotype changes that influence how a gene is read. The result can affect how proteins might be produced, or how many are produced, yet the gene itself does not change. Exposures today can changes how genes are expressed, which can be passed down to grandchildren and future generations.[12,13]

The Endocrine Society has issued precautions about endocrine-disrupting chemicals (EDCs), "It is now well established that developmental exposure to EDCs can alter the epigenome of offspring, affecting gene expression and organogenesis."[14] This equates to significant burden of disease and cost to the health care system: EDCs including flame retardants, pesticides and phthalates are estimated to cost the US $340 billion annually due to IQ loss, infertility, fibroids, endometriosis, and other diseases.[15]

Protecting patients from hazardous exposures before conception is important, because we know that levels can persist in the bodies of the parents, which can have lasting effects on the health of the child long after the parental exposure has been removed.[16] In addition, evidence linking cancers to environmental exposures continues to grow.[17] To effect societal changes, the same general message should be delivered to all patients, as families are important drivers of social norms.

HEALTH PROFESSIONAL AND MEDICAL SOCIETY CONSENSUS STATEMENTS

Scientific consensus among a group of expert toxicologists, health professionals, and patient advocates, called Project TENDR, identified 6 toxic chemical exposures that may contribute to neurodevelopmental disorders including learning disabilities, attention deficit hyperactivity disorder, autism, and behavioral or intellectual impairment.[18] These exposures include: organophosphate pesticides, polybrominated diphenyl ether (PBDE) flame retardants, combustion-related air pollutants, lead, mercury, and polychlorinated biphenyls (PCBs) (often used in carbonless copy paper).[18] Examples of common household or workplace exposures to these chemicals are listed in **Table 1**. In addition, the chemical group phthalates have been highlighted as chemicals of concern due to their activity as EDCs. This endocrine disruption can mimic estrogen, androgens, and other hormonal effects, which may increase the risk of neurodevelopmental disorders, infertility, breast cancer, and prostate cancer.[14,19]

In addition, a coalition of professional medical societies has been organized to highlight the hazardous effects of climate change on human health. This Medical Society Consortium on Climate and Health represents nearly 500,000 physicians, approximately half of US physicians, including the ACOG, the American Academy of Pediatrics, and the American Medical Association. In particular this consortium has identified air pollution as a risk factor for preterm birth and low birth weight.[72]

CLINICAL COUNSELING

Obstetrician-gynecologists and women's health providers play a critical role in educating women about how best to protect their pregnancy from harm. In many cases the clinical visit can be used as the primary intervention for patients to learn about toxic exposure risk assessment and exposure reduction. Many of the opportunities for counseling occur during standard elements of prenatal and preconception care on topics such as food-related exposures, personal care products, and lifestyle modification (ACOG Committee Opinion).

As clinicians, it is most comfortable to discuss topics when there are concrete actions that can be recommended. We are accustomed to double-blinded randomized controlled trials to help us do this when it comes to recommending pharmaceutical treatments. Unlike pharmaceuticals, chemicals have been able to enter our communities with limited or no assessment on their toxicity.[73] The precautionary principle is used by policy makers to justify discretionary decisions in situations where there is the possibility of harm from making a certain decision (eg, taking a particular course of action) when extensive scientific knowledge on the matter is lacking. The principle implies that there is a social responsibility to protect the public from exposure to harm, when scientific investigation has found a plausible risk. These protections can be relaxed only if further scientific findings emerge that provide sound evidence that no harm will result. As a result, the precautionary principle should prevail when it comes to maintaining our ability to reproduce, avoiding neurodevelopmental problems and birth defects in our progeny, and avoiding cancers. Given the potential generational impact, this may be the most important conversation we can have with our patients.

Women's health providers do not need to be experts in environmental health science to provide useful information to patients and refer patients to appropriate specialists when a hazardous exposure is identified. Existing clinical experience and expertise in communicating risks of treatment are largely transferable to environmental health. Physician contact time with a patient does not need to be the primary point of intervention; information and resources about environmental hazards can be successfully incorporated into a childbirth class curriculum or provided in written materials to help parents make optimal choices for themselves and their families.[74,75]

Environmental contaminants can be divided into categories to assist with organizing the information. The impact of exposure depends on external factors such as route, dose, frequency, and timing, as well as factors impacting the susceptibility of the individual such as genetics, epigenetics, age, stage in development, nutritional status, BMI, smoking status, health behaviors, and psychosocial stressors.[76,77] The

Table 1
Environmental exposures, health associations, and clinical counseling

Toxicant	Where Found	Associations	To Minimize Exposure
Lead	House dust, paint, water, soil, imported herbal remedies, cosmetics, jewelry, candy	Miscarriage[20] Lowered intelligence,[21] attention deficits, and behavioral problems[22,23]	Frequently use a wet cloth or mop to clean Look for lead free products
Mercury	Large fish, coal-fired power plants	Decreased cognitive function, decrements in memory,[24,25]	Eat fish with lower levels of mercury Use trusted sites to find local fish advisories http://www.fda.gov/fishadvice https://fishadv.soryonline.epa.gov/General.aspx
Pesticides	Produce, animal products, occupational exposures, home pesticides	Childhood cancers[26] Breast cancer[27] Increased susceptibility to testicular cancer[28] Impaired fetal growth[29] Autism spectrum disorders[30] Decreased intelligence quotient and Decreased working memory[31,32] Poor sperm quality[33]	Eat organic when possible See Environmental Working Group's (EWG's) dirty dozen if unable to choose organic for all foods https://www.ewg.org/foodnews/dirty-dozen.php Avoid using pesticides at home Remove shoes at the door Wash contaminated clothes separately Limit foods high in animal fat. Eat organic dairy products or grass-fed meat sparingly Pets: avoid chemical tick and flea collars, or dips https://prhe.ucsf.edu
Phthalates	Plastics, toys, cleaning and building materials, personal care products, cosmetics and perfumes	Preterm birth,[34,35] attention deficit hyperactivity disorder[36] Hypospadias, undescended testes[37] Neurodevelopmental impairment[38]	Use fragrance-free products rather than fragranced or "unscented" products See EWG site for safe personal care products https://www.ewg.org/consumer-guides Eat fresh organic foods not prepared in plastics

Exposure	Sources	Health effects	Recommendations
Bisphenol A (BPA)	Plastics, liners of canned foods, plastic beverage containers, dental sealants, flooring, paints	Infertility, poor sperm quality[33] PCOS[33,39] and miscarriage[33,40]	Eat fresh organic foods Drink from glass or stainless-steel bottles Avoid microwaving or storing food in plastic containers Reduce the use of canned foods Use BPA-free baby bottles Check recycle codes, those with 3 or 7 may contain BPA
Polychlorinated biphenyls (PCBs)	Foods, bottom-feeding fish, meats, dairy products banned in the 1970s yet persist	Decreased IQ and cognitive functioning[41–43] Increased BMI[44] Decreased semen quality[45] Autism spectrum disorder[46] Breast cancer[47]	Reduce animal fat in your diet Check local fish advisories, choose wild salmon rather than farm-raised salmon
Polybrominated diphenyl ether (PBDE) Flame retardants	House dust, old foam furniture (especially with exposed foam), plastics for electronics	Thyroid disease[48] Decreased fine motor abilities[49] Decrease in cognitive and motor function including lower IQ[49,50]	Choose foam products labeled "flame retardant free" or "compliant with TB-1172013"
Polycyclic aromatic hydrocarbons (PAHs) Air pollution	Released from burning coal, oil, gasoline, wood, cigarette smoking, grilled meats, water contaminated by emissions, vehicle exhaust	Preterm birth[40,51] Low birth weight[52–54] Fetal loss[55,56] Neural tube birth defects[57] Cardiac birth defects[58,59] Asthma[60–63] Allergies[62–65] Cancer[66]	Heed air quality alerts and stay indoors when air quality is poor Avoid cigarette smoke and smoking Support efforts to increase distance from freeways to residential areas Avoid cooking over an open flame when possible
Solvents	Manufacturing, dry cleaning, printing, stain removers, paint thinners, nail polish removers, insulation, fiberglass	Miscarriage[67,68] Low birth weight[69,70] Cardiac birth defects[71]	Limit use Ensure in a well-ventilated area with protection of the skin when used

information in **Table 1** is presented as a guide for general discussion regarding exposures that can be hazardous, where they are encountered in our communities, associated outcomes published about chemicals in the class, and reasonable strategies for decreasing exposure.

SPECIFIC TOXICANTS

Lead bioaccumulates in the bone and is mobilized during pregnancy due to high calcium turnover. It is neurotoxic to a developing fetus, and exposure can result in lowered intelligence. Intellectual deficits, attention deficits, impulsivity, aggression, and hyperactivity occur with even lower levels of lead exposure.[21,78]

If risk factors are present, consider blood testing of lead levels. For advice on testing or chelation, reach out to your local poison control center (www.aapcc.org/dnn/AAPCC/FindLocalPoisonCenters.aspx) or an environmental medicine expert (www.aoec.org).

Widespread poisoning with methylmercury-contaminated seafood occurred in the Minamata area of Japan as a byproduct of a manufacturing process that began in the 1950s. Symptoms of methylmercury poisoning include sensory disturbances, muscle weakness, ataxia, visual field changes, articulation disorders, hearing loss, and death. Fetuses can experience mental retardation, inability to walk, disturbances of coordination, speech, chewing and swallowing, and increased muscle tone, similar to cerebral palsy. This can occur in the absence of symptoms in the mother, consistent with the findings that methylmercury accumulates in the fetus,[79,80] and that the fetal brain is particularly sensitive to methylmercury.[81] Prenatal exposures to low levels of mercury can have a long-lasting impact on childhood psychomotor development.[74] It took over a decade to recognize the environmental issue, because the inclination was to initially think that an unidentified infectious agent was the cause.[81]

Pesticides are a diverse group of chemicals that are used in large quantities in agricultural settings and, as such, contaminate our water, food, air, and soil. They can be inhaled, absorbed via the skin, and ingested. Some have been implicated in impaired fetal growth, cognitive development, and neurodevelopment with *in utero* exposure. There are increased risks of cancer with some exposures during childhood and later in life. It is recommended to use nonchemical methods of controlling pests or to prevent pests from coming into the home or garden. Fixing leaks, sealing cracks, clearing the yard of overgrown brush or objects that can hold standing water can help. When needed, the use of mechanical traps decreases the need to use chemicals. Organic farming or gardening provides an alternative to the use of synthetic pesticides by using soil management, crop rotation, companion planting, and fostering predator insects to deal with pests.

Phthalates are chemicals added to make plastics more flexible, transparent, and durable. They can also be found in personal care products such as cosmetics, soap, lotions, and shampoo. They have been found in urine, serum, amniotic fluid, and breast milk,[82] and have been associated with birth defects, neurodevelopmental impairment, and preterm birth.[34–38] Products should be sought that are labeled "fragrance free" or "scented with only essential oils." Bisphenol A (BPA) is a material used to make plastic containers to store food and beverages, resins that line pipes, as well as thermal paper. The National Institute of Environmental Health Sciences, part of the NIH, advises against heating plastic food containers as they may break down over time. This allows chemicals such as BPA to leach into food. Instead use glass, porcelain or stainless-steel containers. When using plastics look for recycle codes 1, 2, or 5, because containers with recycle codes 3 or 7 may contain BPA and/or phthalates.

PCBs were initially used for insulating electrical equipment and for other industrial purposes. Their hazards to health were demonstrated, and, since 1970, PCBs have been banned in the United States; however, they are quite persistent in the environment and are increased as one moves up the food chain. At this point our largest exposures come from bottom-feeding fish, meats, and dairy products. Striped bass, bluefish, American eel, and sea trout are bottom feeders, and larger predator fish such as bass, lake trout, and walleye from contaminated waters can also have higher levels of PCBs, which concentrate in fat. Many farm-raised salmon are fed ground up small fish in which PCBs can be concentrated, wild salmon often have lower levels. The US EPA recommends removing the skin fat and internal organs before fish is cooked.[83] Increasing exposure has been associated with decreased IQ and decreased cognitive functioning in multiple studies, even since the ban.[41–43] Reducing animal fat in the diet is the best means of decreasing exposure.

The California fires created concern in the 1970s. In 1975, the CA legislature passed a law requiring all seating furniture sold in the state to be flame retardant. CA technical bulletin 117 (TB 117) [84] spelled out the specifics. Given that California was the 12th largest economy in the world, this resulted in flame retardants (including PBDEs) being put into consumer products worldwide. Unfortunately, flame retardants have not helped to impact fire-related deaths. Although attempts to ban flame retardants has been unsuccessful in California, on September 30, 2014, Governor Brown signed into law SB1019 (Leno) requiring labeling regarding the presence of flame retardants, and there have been substantive changes to TB 117, which no longer specifies conditions requiring chemical intervention. PBDEs disrupt the endocrine systems of humans both during development and throughout the lifespan; thyroid disease most strongly correlates to women exposed during menopause.[48]

Polycyclic aromatic hydrocarbons (PAHs) are a group of at least 100 chemicals released from burning oil, coal, gasoline, wood, tobacco, and trash. Particulate matter is a mixture of liquid droplets and solid particles found in the air. Air pollution and particulate matter have been shown to be associated with preterm birth,[51,52] low birth weight,[52–54] fetal loss,[55,56] cardiac,[58,59] and neural tube birth defects,[57] and have been labeled by the International Agency for Research on Cancer to be carcinogenic in humans.[66]

Solvents are broadly used in various industries for cleaning, painting, refinishing, embalming, and degreasing. They are commonly found in the home in automotive products, varnishes, nail polish, thinners, and stain removers. Tetrachloroethylene commonly used in dry cleaning has been shown to be associated with miscarriages. Benzene and trichloroethylene are known carcinogens. Toluene, commonly used in print-based media, is associated with decreased fetal birth weight.[85] Solvents are typically inhaled or absorbed through the skin. Avoidance when possible is recommended, and they should be used in a well-ventilated area with gloves and eye protection when they must be used.

A simple questionnaire should be considered (**Table 2**) at routine gynecology, preconception, initial prenatal, and postpartum visits. The questionnaire should be set up so that a positive response would trigger the provision of information. For example, if a patient indicates a diet rich in fish, recommending checking the EPA's site to find local fish advisories that can help limit exposure to mercury and PCBs. Because some of the effects can affect health not only for a developing fetus, but for adults as well, the advice is pertinent beyond pregnancy-related visits. Some targeted advice can be found in the last column of **Table 1**.

Table 2
Sample environmental health questionnaire

Question			Pertains to
Do you live in a home built before 1970?	[ ] Yes	[ ] No	Lead
Do you purchase imported goods such as: cosmetics, herbal remedies, or candy?	[ ] Yes	[ ] No	Lead
Do you crave and chew ice cubes daily?	[ ] Yes	[ ] No	Lead
Do you make or use lead-glazed pottery?	[ ] Yes	[ ] No	Lead
Do you work or live near a coal-fired power plant?	[ ] Yes	[ ] No	Mercury, PAHs
Do you eat fish or shellfish more than 3 times per week?	[ ] Yes	[ ] No	Mercury, PCBs
Do you work with pesticides?	[ ] Yes	[ ] No	Pesticides
Do you use pesticides or insecticides for the lawn or garden?	[ ] Yes	[ ] No	Pesticides
Do you use chemical flea preparations, flea collars, or flea dips for your pet?	[ ] Yes	[ ] No	Pesticides
Do you use plastic containers to microwave or store food?	[ ] Yes	[ ] No	Phthalates, BPA
Do you work with solvents (adhesives, varnishes, thinners, automotive products, degreasers) on a regular basis?	[ ] Yes	[ ] No	Solvents
Do you use fragranced personal care products (perfumes, lotions, and deodorants)?	[ ] Yes	[ ] No	Phthalates
Do you eat meat or consume dairy products most days each week?	[ ] Yes	[ ] No	Pesticides, PCBs
Do you have furniture purchased before 2014 with exposed foam?	[ ] Yes	[ ] No	PBDEs
Do you live near a high-traffic area?	[ ] Yes	[ ] No	PAH's
Do you cook over an open flame or have an open-air fireplace?	[ ] Yes	[ ] No	PAHs
Do you eat canned foods?	[ ] Yes	[ ] No	BPA
Do you drink from plastic bottles?	[ ] Yes	[ ] No	BPA
Do you work with flooring, dental sealants or paint?	[ ] Yes	[ ] No	BPA

SUMMARY

There is no perfect way to avoid every exposure. We make the best decisions we can with the information readily available to us at any given time. Clinically, discussions with patients focused on prevention of future exposures rather than on past exposures and possible implications may be most productive.

Although each of us can do his or her best to avoid harmful toxicants, prevention really requires support on a societal level. For market forces to drive change, broad understanding is needed, including educating our patients with regard to toxicants exposure, the impacts they may have, and transparency with regard to ingredients in every product sold. A good first start is focusing on labeling requirements, which is generally accomplished by legislation or regulation.

The involvement and support from organized medicine and local medical societies is crucial. As individual health care providers, our patients trust us to provide sound guidance when it comes to preventing disease and impacting disease susceptibility for future generations. On a broader level women's health providers can help by supporting efforts to require manufacturers to ensure safety before introducing new chemicals into our environment and to evaluate the safety of those already present.

REFERENCES

1. American College of Obstetricians and Gynecologists. American College of Obstetricians and Gynecologists: committee opinion 575. Exposure to toxic environmental agents. Washington (DC): American College of Obstetricians and Gynecologists; 2013.
2. Di Renzo G, Conry JA, Blake J, et al. International Federation of Gynecology and Obstetrics opinion on reproductive health impacts of exposure to toxic environmental chemicals. Int J Gynaecol Obstet 2015;131:219–25.
3. United States Environmental Protection Agency. Assessing and managing chemicals under TSCA 2017. Available at: https://www.epa.gov/assessing-and-managing-chemicals-under-tsca/frank-r-lautenberg-chemical-safety-21st-century-act. Accessed December 26, 2018.
4. United States Environmental Protection Agency. TSCA chemical substance inventory. 2016. Available at: https://www.epa.gov/tsca-inventory/about-tsca-chemical-substance-inventory#whatistheinventory. Accessed December 26, 2018.
5. United States Environmental Protection Agency. EPA takes first steps in identifying next group of chemicals for risk evaluation under TSCA 2018. Available at: https://www.epa.gov/newsreleases/epa-takes-first-steps-identifying-next-group-chemicals-risk-evaluation-under-tsca. Accessed December 26, 2018.
6. Woodruff TJ, Sutton P. Practitioner insights: the peril and imperative of TSCA reform. Bloomberg BNA environment and energy report 2017.
7. Krimsky M, Forster DE, Llabre MM, et al. The influence of time on task on mind wandering and visual working memory. Cognition 2017;169:84–90.
8. Maffini MV, Neltner TG, Vogel S. We are what we eat: regulatory gaps in the United States that put our health at risk. Biology 2017;15(12):1–8.
9. DeNicola N, Zlatnik M, Conry J. Toxic environmental exposures in maternal, fetal, and reproductive health. Contemp Ob Gyn 2018.
10. Woodruff TJ, Zota AR, Schwartz JM. Environmental chemicals in pregnant women in the United States: NHANES 2003–2004. Environ Health Perspect 2011;119(6):878–85.

11. Wang A, Gerona RR, Schwartz JM, et al. A suspect screening method for characterizing multiple chemical exposures among a demographically diverse population of pregnant women in San Francisco. Environ Health Perspect 2018;126(7): 077009.

12. Iguchi T, Miyagawa S, Sudo T. Modern genetics of reproductive biology. In: Woodruff TJ, Janssen SJ, Guillette LJ Jr, et al, editors. Environmental impacts on reproductive health and fertility. New York: Cambridge University Press; 2010. p. 60–71.

13. Grandjean P, Bellinger D, Bergman A, et al. The Faroes statement: human health effects of developmental exposure to chemicals in our environment. Basic Clin Pharmacol Toxicol 2008;102:73–5.

14. The Endocrine Society. Position statement: endocrine-disrupting chemicals 2018. Available at: https://www.endocrine.org/-/media/endosociety/files/advocacy-and-outreach/position-statements/2018/position_statement_endocrine_disrupting_chemicals.pdf?la=en.

15. Attina TM, Hauser R, Sathyanarayana S, et al. Exposure to endocrine-disrupting chemicals in the USA: a population-based disease burden and cost analysis. Lancet Diabetes Endocrinol 2016;8587(16):1–8.

16. Grason H, Misra D. Reducing exposure to environmental toxicants before birth: moving from risk perception to risk reduction. Public Health Rep 2009;124(5): 629–41.

17. National Cancer Institute. Reducing environmental cancer risk: what we can do now. President's cancer panel 2008–2009 annual report. Bethesda (MD): NCI; 2010. Available at: http://deainfo.nci.nih.gov/advisory/pcp/annualReports/pcp08-09rpt/PCP_Report_08-09_508.pdf. Accessed December 24, 2018.

18. Bennett D, Bellinger DC, Birnbaum LS, et al. Project TENDR: targeting environmental neuro-developmental risks the TENDR consensus statement. Environ Health Perspect 2016;124(7):118–22.

19. DeNicola N, Zlatnik MG, Conry J. Toxic environmental exposures in maternal, fetal, and reproductive health. Contemp Ob Gyn 2018;63(9):34–8.

20. Slama R, Cordier S. Environmental contaminants and impacts on healthy and successful pregnancies. In: Woodruff TJ, Janssen SJ, Guillette LJ Jr, et al, editors. Environmental impacts on reproductive health and fertility. New York: Cambridge University Press; 2010. p. 125–44.

21. Lanphear BP, Hornung R, Khoury J, et al. Low-level environmental lead exposure and children's intellectual function:an international pooled analysis. Environ Health Perspect 2005;113(7):894–9.

22. Eubig PA, Aguiar A, Schantz SL. Lead and PCBs as risk factors for attention deficit/hyperactivity disorder. Environ Health Perspect 2010;118(12):1654–67.

23. Council on Environmental Health. Prevention of childhood lead toxicity. Pediatrics 2016;138(1):e20161493.

24. Debes F, Budtz-Jorgensen E, Weihe P, et al. Impact of prenatal methylmercury exposure on neurobehavioral function at age 14 years. Neurotoxicol Teratol 2006;28:536–47.

25. Orenstein ST, Thurston SW, Bellinger DC, et al. Prenatal organochlorine and methylmercury exposure and memory and learning in school-age children in communities near the New Bedford Harbor Superfund site, Massachusetts. Environ Health Perspect 2014;122(11):1253–9.

26. Wigle DT, Turner MC, Krewski D. A systematic review and meta-analysis of childhood leukemia and parental occupational pesticide exposure. Environ Health Perspect 2009;117:1505–13.

27. Gray J, Rasanayagam S, Engel C, et al. State of the evidence 2017: an update on the connection between breast cancer and the environment. Environ Health 2017;16:94.

28. Cohn BA, Cirillo PM, Christianson RE. Prenatal DDT exposure and testicular cancer: a nested case-control study. Arch Environ Occup Health 2010;65:127–34.

29. Whyatt RM, Rauh V, Barr D, et al. Prenatal insecticide exposures and birth weight and length among an urban minority cohort. Environ Health Perspect 2004;112: 1125–32.

30. Rauh VA, Garfinkel R, Perera FP, et al. Impact of prenatal chlorpyrifos exposure on neurodevelopment in the first 3 years of life among inner-city children. Pediatrics 2006;118:1845–59.

31. Bouchard MF, Chevrier J, Harley K, et al. Prenatal exposure to organophosphate pesticides and IQ in 7-year-old children. Environ Health Perspect 2011;119: 1189–95.

32. Rauh V, Arunajadai S, Horton M, et al. Seven-year neurodevelopmental scores and prenatal exposure to chlorpyrifos, a common agricultural pesticide. Environ Health Perspect 2011;119:1196–201.

33. Stavros S, Androutsopoulos VP, Tsatsakis AM, et al. Human exposure to endocrine disrupting chemicals: effects on the male and female reproductive systems. Environ Toxicol Pharmacol 2017;51:56–70.

34. Ferguson KK, McElrath TF, Meeker JD. Environmental phthalate exposure and preterm birth. JAMA Pediatr 2014;168(1):61–7.

35. Ferguson KK, Chen YH, Tyler J, et al. Mediation of the relationship between maternal phthalate exposure and preterm birth by oxidative stress with repeated measurements across pregnancy. Environ Health Perspect 2017;125(3):488–94.

36. Engel SM, Miodovnik A, Canfield RL, et al. Prenatal phthalate exposure is associated with childhood behaviour and executive functioning. Environ Health Perspect 2010;118:565–71.

37. Salma, 2010.

38. Engel SM, Zhu C, Berkowitz GS, et al. Prenatal phthalate exposure and performance on the neonatal behavioral assessment scale in a multiethnic birth cohort. Neruotoxicology 2009;30:522–8.

39. Rutkowska, 2016.

40. Sugiura-Ogasawara M, Yasuhiko O, Tamao K. Diagnosis and treatment methods for recurrent miscarriage cases. Reprod Med Biol 2009;8(4):141–4.

41. Jacobson JL, Jacobson SW. Intellectual impairment in children exposed to polychlorinated biphenyls in utero. N Engl J Med 1996;335(11):783–9.

42. Jacobson J. Effects of in utero exposure to polychlorinated biphenyls and related contaminants on cognitive functioning in young children. J Pediatr 1990;116(1): 38–45.

43. Stewart PW, Lonky E, Reihman J, et al. The relationship between prenatal PCB exposure and intelligence (IQ) in 9-year old children. Environ Health Perspect 2008;116(10):1416–22.

44. Verhust SL, Nelen V, Hond ED, et al. Intrauterine exposure to environmental pollutants and body mass index during the first 3 years of life. Environ Health Perspect 2009;117:122–6.

45. Dallinga JW. Decreased human semen quality and organochlorine compounds in blood. Hum Reprod 2002;17:1973–9.

46. Lyall K, Croen L, Sjodin A, et al. Polychlorinated biphenyl and organochlorine pesticide concentrations in maternal mid-pregnancy serum samples: association

with autism spectrum disorder and intellectual disability. Environ Health Perspect 2017;125(3):474–80.

47. Pastor-Barriuso R, Fernandez MF, Castano-Vinyals G, et al. Total effective xenoestrogen burden in serum samples and risk for breast cancer in a population-based multicase-control study in Spain. Environ Health Perspect 2016;124(10):1575–82.

48. Allen J, Gale S, Zoeller RT, et al. PBDE flame retardants, thyroid disease, and menopausal status in U.S. women. Environ Health 2016;15:60.

49. Roze E, Meijer L, Bakker A, et al. Prenatal exposure to organohalogens, including brominated flame retardants, influences motor, cognitive and behavioral performance at school age. Environ Health Perspect 2009;117(12):1953–8.

50. Herbstman JB, Sjodin A, Kurzon, et al. Prenatal exposure to PBDEs and neurodevelopment. Environ Health Perspect 2010;118:712–9.

51. Chang HH, Reich BJ, Miranda ML. Time-to-event analysis of fine particle air pollution and preterm birth: results from North Carolina, 2001–2005. Am J Epidemiol 2012;175(2):91–8.

52. Wilhelm M, Ritz B. Local variations in CO and particulate air pollution and adverse birth outcomes in Los Angeles County, California, USA. Environ Health Perspect 2005;113(9):1212–21.

53. Dadvand P, Parker J, Bell ML, et al. Maternal exposure to particulate air pollution and term birth weight: a multi-country evaluation of effect and heterogeneity. Environ Health Perspect 2013;121(3):267–373.

54. Rich DQ, Lui K, Zhang J, et al. Differences in birth weight associated with the 2008 Beijing Olympic air pollution reduction: results from a natural experiment. Environ Health Perspect 2015;123(9):880–7.

55. Hou HY, Wang D, Zou XP, et al. Does ambient air pollutants increase the risk of fetal loss? A case-control study. Arch Gynecol Obstet 2014;289(2):285–91.

56. Ha S, Sundaram R, Buck Louis GM, et al. Ambient air pollution and the risk of pregnancy loss: a prospective cohort study. Fertil Steril 2018;109(1):148–53.

57. Padula AM, Tager IB, Carmichael SL, et al. The association of ambient air pollution and traffic exposures with selected congenital anomalies in the San Joaquin Valley of California. Am J Epidemiol 2013;177(10):1074–85.

58. Ritz B, Yu F, Fruin S, et al. Ambient air pollution and risk of birth defects in southern California. Am J Epidemiol 2002;155(1):17–25.

59. Gilboa SM, Mendola P, Olshan AF, et al. Relation between ambient air quality and selected birth defects, seven county study, Texas, 1997–2000. Am J Epidemiol 2005;162:238–52.

60. Hsu HH, Chiu YH, Coull BA, et al. Prenatal particulate air pollution and asthma onset in urban children. Identifying sensitive windows and sex differences. Am J Respir Crit Care Med 2015;192:1052–9.

61. Nishimura KK, Galanter JM, Roth LA, et al. Early-life air pollution and asthma risk in minority children. The GALA II and SAGE II studies. Am J Respir Crit Care Med 2013;188:309–18.

62. Gehring U, Wijga AH, Brauer M, et al. Traffic-related air pollution and the development of asthma and allergies during the first 8 years of life. Am J Respir Crit Care Med 2010;181:596–603.

63. Bowatte G, Lodge C, Lowe AJ, et al. The influence of childhood traffic-related air pollution exposure on asthma, allergy and sensitization: a systematic review and a meta-analysis of birth cohort studies. Allergy 2015;70:245–56.

64. Sbihi H, Allen RW, Becker A, et al. Perinatal exposure to traffic-related air pollution and atopy at 1 year of age in a multi-center Canadian birth cohort study. Environ Health Perspect 2015;123:902–8.

65. Morales E, Garcia-Esteban R, de la Cruz OA, et al. Intrauterine and early post-natal exposure to outdoor air pollution and lung function at preschool age. Thorax 2015;70:64–73.

66. International Agency for Research on Cancer. Outdoor air pollution. IARC Monogr Eval Carcinog Risks Hum 2013;109:1–454. Available at: https://monographs.iarc. fr/ENG/Monographs/vol109/mono109-F01.pdf. Accessed January 1, 2019.

67. Hruska KS, Furth PA, Seifer DB, et al. Environmental factors in infertility. Clin Obstet Gynecol 2000;43(4):821–9.

68. Kyyronen P, Taskinen H, Lindbohm ML, et al. Spontaneous abortions and congenital malformations among women exposed to tetrachloroethylene in dry cleaning. J Epidemiol Community Health 1989;43(4):346–51.

69. Vaktskjold A, Talykova LV, Nieboert E. Low birth weight in newborns to women employed in jobs with frequent exposure to organic solvents. Int J Environ Health Res 2014;24(1):44–55.

70. Ahmed P, Jaakkola JJ. Exposure to organic solvents and adverse pregnancy outcomes. Hum Reprod 2007;22:2751–7.

71. Makris SL, Scott CS, Fox J, et al. Review: a systematic evaluation of the potential effects of trichlorethylene exposure on cardiac development. Reprod Toxicol 2016;65:321–58.

72. Medical Society Consortium on Climate and Health. Medical alert! Climate change is harming our health 2017. Available at: https://medsocietiesforclimatehealth.org/wp-content/uploads/2017/03/gmu_medical_alert_updated_082417.pdf.

73. Wang A, Padula A, Sirota M, et al. Environmental influences on reproductive health: the importance of chemical exposures. Fertil Steril 2016;106(4):905–29.

74. Tatsuta N, Nakai K, Sakamoto M, et al. Methylmercury exposure and developmental outcomes in Tohoku study of child development at 18 months of age. Toxics 2018;6(3):49.

75. ACO CO.

76. Woodruff TJ, Giudice LC. Introduction. In: Woodruff TJ, Janssen SJ, Guillette LJ Jr, et al, editors. Environmental impacts on reproductive health and fertility. New York: Cambridge University Press; 2010. p. 1–7.

77. Lanphear BP. The impact of toxins on the developing brain. Annu Rev Public Health 2015;36:211–30.

78. National Toxicology Program.

79. Rollin HB, Rudge CV, Thomassen Y, et al. Levels of toxic and essential metals in maternal and umbilical cord blood from selected areas of South Africa - results of a pilot study. J Environ Monit 2009;11:618–27.

80. Stern AH, Smith AE. An assessment of the cord blood: maternal blood methylmercury ratio: implications for risk assessment. Environ Health Perspect 2003;111:1465–70.

81. Sakamoto M, Tatsuta N, Izumo K, et al. Health impacts and biomarkers of prenatal exposure to methylmercury: lessons from Minamata, Japan. Toxics 2018;6(3):45.

82. Fox MA, Aoki Y. Environmental contaminants and exposure. In: Woodruff TJ, Janssen SJ, Guillette LJ Jr, et al, editors. Environmental impacts on reproductive health and fertility. New York: Cambridge University Press; 2010. p. 8–22.

83. United States Environmental Protection Agency. Should I eat the fish I catch? 2014. Available at: https://www.epa.gov/sites/production/files/2015-07/documents/english_updated_fishbrochure.pdf. Accessed December 31, 2018.

84. State of California. Technical bulletin 117: requirements, test procedure, and apparatus for testing the flame retardance of resilient filling materials used in upholstered furniture. North Highlands (CA): Bureau of Home Furnishings and Thermal Insulation; 2000.

85. Donald JM, Hooper K, Hopenhayan-Rich C. Reproductive and developmental toxicity of toluene: a review. Environ Health Perspect 1991;94:237–44.

Integrated Mind/Body Care in Women's Health

A Focus on Well-Being, Mental Health, and Relationships

Priya Batra, PsyD

KEYWORDS

- Integrated health care • Women's health psychology
- Psychological concerns in OB/GYN • Well-being in women's health

KEY POINTS

- The presentation of psychological concerns in primary care departments is common and inadequately being addressed in the current systems of care.
- Inclusion of mental health clinicians in the same department as medical providers improves detection of and intervention for psychosocial conditions.
- Reduction of stigma around psychological conditions and care is possible with integrated care and has been shown to be a satisfier for health care providers and patients.
- Addressing relationship concerns via new models of integrated health care can improve overall health for the patient and her family.

It has been said that if you build it, they will come. Sometimes it takes the alternative, demand it and it will be built, for systems to evolve and meet consumer needs in an obvious, but paradigm-shifting manner. We are now solidly in the fifth wave of public health, the era of well-being. The first four waves included: public works, germ theory, institution restructuring, and lifestyle risk.[1] Although the work around risk reduction and disease management will never truly be over, medical and technological advancements have allowed us to now give needed attention to the social and emotional roots of well-being. Knowledge of patients' developmental milestones and adversities, coupled with the buffers of resilience and healthy relationships over the lifespan, will move us toward better understanding of the mind/body connection and holistic healing. This requires facility with strategies that foster behavioral change and use of the relational alliance between provider and patient to achieve progress, satisfaction, and overall health. It was controversial in 1946

Disclosure Statement: The author has nothing to disclose.
Kaiser Permanente, Women's Health, 1650 Response Road, Sacramento, CA 95815, USA
E-mail address: priya.x.batra@kp.org

when the World Health Organization asserted in their constitution that "health is a state of complete physical, mental, and social well-being and not merely the absence of disease or infirmity."[2] Seventy plus years later, health care institutions around the globe still strive to make this vision a part of daily practice. Achievement of true mind/body health and provision of holistic care requires multidisciplinary perspectives and a team of interconnected professionals to offer diversified health care services, ideally in shared spaces.

Having highly trained mental health clinicians embedded in primary care units is how more women can have their psychological and behavioral health needs met in a nonstigmatizing and naturalistic manner. While in their health care home, patients can speak with their "body doctors" and "feelings doctors" within the same arena and ostensibly, with the same level of importance given to all raised health concerns. This is the job that this author has been doing for 17 years and how it is simplistically described to her 7-year-old daughter. Almost without fail, quizzical looks appear when the title "women's health psychologist" is shared. The understanding is palpable, however, when it is explained that mood and anxiety conditions are the number one cause of maternal health complications during and after pregnancy,[3] that times of hormonal transition (eg, menarche, puberty, menstrual complications, pregnancy and matrescence,[4] breastfeeding, perimenopause, and menopause) are also times of psychological vulnerability, and that obstetrical and gynecological (OB/GYN) challenges (eg, infertility, unplanned pregnancy, pregnancy loss, myriad pregnancy complications, pelvic pain, sexual functioning concerns, gynecologic cancers) impact physical and emotional well-being and should be treated beyond just the medical symptom presentation. Rarely is there push-back when it is noted that relational aggression, most often in the forms of domestic violence and sexual violations, is all too frequently brought up by OB/GYN patients and that the frontline medical providers do not have the adequate time to hear out their patients' stories and then respond with behavioral and psychological recommendations that can guide such patients on their paths toward understanding the impact of what occurred and then moving toward healing.

The time is now to advance the practice of mind/body medicine and to have mental health professionals working alongside their medical colleagues. The American Psychological Association released "Briefing Series on the Role of Psychology in Health Care"[5] in 2014 and a video in 2015 entitled "Psychologists in Integrated Health Care: Obstetrics and Gynecology."[6] Unfortunately, the integration recommended and displayed in these two resources is still the exception rather than common place and much work is needed to advance this vision of mind/body care. Poleshuck and Woods[7] heralded a similar call in 2014 and this paper seeks to further advance their call for patient-centered models of health care delivery in women's health departments. An American College of Obstetricians and Gynecologists[8] review of published studies between 2005 and 2009 found that OB/GYN providers were more adept at screening for depression than anxiety. They also believed that time and skill limitations affected what mental health issues they could be helpful with; they were twice as often treating with antidepressants rather than referring to mental health professionals. Another study[9] found that obstetric women's health patients are more than four times likely to pursue psychological treatment when they can receive such services at the same site as their women's health provider; in fact, it was the most robust predictor of treatment attendance of all the factors examined. This same study highlighted the need for embedded mental health workers and noted that the unmet need for psychiatric care in their perinatal population was 48%. The data are present, now the will must be activated.

WHAT IS WELL-BEING?

Well-being is a much-used but not always well-defined concept. Different professions prioritize various aspects of well-being and therefore may measure the constructs of well-being via different tools. A recent analysis[10] of self-report assessments of well-being found that the existing tools of measurement tended to revolve around six themes: (1) mental well-being, (2) social well-being, (3) physical well-being, (4) spiritual well-being, (5) personal circumstances, and (6) activities and functioning. Gallup scientists have asserted that the five elements of well-being include (1) career well-being, (2) social well-being, (3) financial well-being, (4) physical well-being, and (5) community well-being.[11] Thriving is only possible when one has a sense of wellness in all five domains. The threshold of suffering varies based on functional ability and safety, self-comparison with previous functioning, and interpersonal comparison. Importantly, when one domain is causing hardship it may bring about loss of capacity or decreased sense of wellness in the other domains. Most medical providers can readily name many clinical examples of patients who repeatedly present for care with a moving target of symptoms, a general sense of malaise, and a lack of clinical findings to explain the symptom presentation. This is where a psychological assessment could prove clarifying for the providers and patients.

THE REFERRAL PROCESS

When primary care departments are not colocated with psychiatry or behavioral health departments, follow through on such referrals by patients tends to be low.[12] It has been said that primary care departments in the United States are actually the centers for de facto mental health care and that this system is fraught with complications, inadequacies, and challenges. Stigma is also not addressed when patients are required to navigate themselves through new departments and systems. Approximately 25% to 30% of inpatient cases have been found to have significant psychiatric components and this number is also similarly high for outpatient visits. Detection, accurate diagnosing, and triaging of these conditions has been found to be poor.[13] Although there is now widespread awareness that perinatal patients should be screened for psychiatric conditions, patient follow through on mental health visits is at 22% if interventions are not readily made available to them and still just at 31% with concerted follow-up and individual and group therapy made available. Rates of mental health engagement are doubled when patient and provider barriers are addressed (ie, patient engagement strategies, on-site assessments, and training of healthcare providers on perinatal mental health issues).[14] The women's health psychologist could take the lead on all these efforts.

Embedment of a mental health clinician within the primary care team or colocation of a mental health provider allows for familiarity between providers. The solidity of the relationship is built on two platforms: trust between professionals and knowledge about scopes of practice. When these foundational elements are present, providers can convey a sense of confidence in the professional who is being suggested and the skill-set of that professional partner. Likewise, communication between providers is made easy and true collaborative care can become part of the normative functioning in the department.

So as not to create a mini psychiatry department within the women's health arena, the focus of the mental health clinician would be on rapid assessment, brief intervention, and triaging for mental health services. Accurate diagnosis is key, as is awareness of the spectrum of services available to patients within the health care system (eg, behavioral health classes and what affiliated departments of psychiatry and/

or behavioral health have to offer for psychotherapy) and in the surrounding communities. Psychologists are capable and skilled at discussing with patients whether a first-line psychotropic (eg, selective serotonin reuptake inhibitors) should be initiated and then convey the patient's openness to trying such medications quickly to the referring provider who then can write a prescription long before the patient may be able to meet with a psychiatrist. Many times, attention to the bottom two tiers of Maslow's hierarchy of needs[15] (ie, physiologic and safety needs) is first required and a service, such as 211,[16] a free informational and referral system, can be discussed with the patient. In California, 96% of the population has access to this service and in the United States overall, that number is 85%. It is tough, if not impossible, to address needs of the psyche if one is from the outset lacking in housing, safety, and basic necessities and resources. The mental health clinician's myriad role in the women's health department can include being an ambassador to community linkages and an educator/supporter of the medical staff around appropriate referrals for various social needs.

The American College of Obstetricians and Gynecologists (ACOG) and the United States Preventive Services Task Force (USPSTF) have published position statements on an array of behavioral health conditions that they recommend be given attention in the primary care arena. The Women's Preventive Services Initiative (WPSI) recommends that screening for depression and intimate partner violence take place at the well-woman visit across a woman's lifespan. Most doctor office visits in OB/GYN clinics are limited to 15 minutes and addressing such complicated and sensitive topics in a comprehensive manner would ideally require partnership and warm hand-off to a colleague specializing in psychological assessment and intervention. The effectiveness of the mental health professional is enhanced when not only social determinants of health[17] are attended to, but diversity issues are as well.[18] So often, the populations who are underserved by the health care system are those who may think that psychological interventions would be unavailable or unhelpful to them. Among this group may be the non-English speaking, recent immigrants, the impoverished, and the disabled. The health care system can aid in debunking such a premise, and in reducing stigma around the acceptance of psychological services, when the psychological care is made easy and flexible to access. As noted, although embedment is one such way to remove barriers to care, the use of telephone consultation and video visits are also viable options. Colocation of services for mind/body care allows for clear assertion of an organization's values around care for the whole person.

Regardless of whether the patient presents in the preconception time period, for a routine OB/GYN visit, for a specific presenting concern, or for prenatal or postpartum care, the psychologist may prove to be an invaluable partner to the health care team. Patients often disclose current psychiatric and social struggles and may not be in a position of connecting the dots between their personal experiences, psychological health, and medical concerns. Without needing to refer to an external department, trust and comfort may be afforded in a more expedient manner when a same-day consultation is available or the referring provider is able to speak confidently and positively about the embedded mental health clinician with whom the patient could meet in the near future (**Table 1**).

PSYCHOLOGICAL SERVICES IN WOMEN'S HEALTH
General Psychosocial Distress

A common scenario for primary care providers is that their patient either has a host of concerns that cannot possibly be adequately addressed in a 15-minute visit or the

Table 1
Behavioral health recommendations (ACOG and USPSTF)

Behavioral Health Focus	Opinion/Recommendation Statements
Alcohol use	ACOG: https://www.acog.org/Clinical-Guidance-and-Publications/Committee-Opinions/Committee-on-Health-Care-for-Underserved-Women/At-Risk-Drinking-and-Alcohol-Dependence-Obstetric-and-Gynecologic-Implications USPSTF: https://www.uspreventiveservicestaskforce.org/Page/Document/RecommendationStatementFinal/alcohol-misuse-screening-and-behavioral-counseling-interventions-in-primary-care
Depression	ACOG: https://www.acog.org/About-ACOG/News-Room/Statements/2016/ACOG-Statement-on-Depression Screening USPSTF: https://www.uspreventiveservicestaskforce.org/Page/Document/RecommendationStatementFinal/depression-in-adults-screening
Drug abuse, dependence, and addiction	ACOG (Toolkit): https://www.acog.org//media/Departments/Government-Relations-and-Outreach/NASToolkit.pdf
Drug use, illicit	USPSTF: https://www.uspreventiveservicestaskforce.org/Page/Document/ClinicalSummaryFinal/drug-use-illicit-screening
Intimate partner violence	ACOG: https://www.acog.org/Clinical-Guidance-and-Publications/Committee-Opinions/Committee-on-Health-Care-for-Underserved-Women/Intimate-Partner-Violence?IsMobileSet=false USPSTF: https://www.uspreventiveservicestaskforce.org/Page/Document/RecommendationStatementFinal/intimate-partner-violence-and-abuse-of-elderly-and-vulnerable-adults-screening1
Methamphetamine use in women of reproductive age	ACOG: https://www.acog.org/Clinical-Guidance-and-Publications/Committee-Opinions/Committee-on-Health-Care-for-Underserved-Women/Methamphetamine-Abuse-in-Women-of-Reproductive-Age
Preconception care	ACOG: https://www.acog.org/Clinical-Guidance-and-Publications/Committee-Opinions/Committee-on-Gynecologic-Practice/The-Importance-of-Preconception-Care-in-the-Continuum-of-Womens-Health-Care
Reproductive and sexual coercion	ACOG: https://www.acog.org/Clinical-Guidance-and-Publications/Committee-Opinions/Committee-on-Health-Care-for-Underserved-Women/Reproductive-and-Sexual-Coercion
Smoking	ACOG (cessation in pregnancy): https://www.acog.org/Clinical-Guidance-and-Publications/Committee-Opinions/Committee-on-Obstetric-Practice/Smoking-Cessation-During-Pregnancy?IsMobileSet=false USPSTF (including pregnant women): https://www.uspreventiveservicestaskforce.org/Page/Document/UpdateSummaryFinal/tobacco-use-in-adults-and-pregnant-women-counseling-and-interventions1

Abbreviations: ACOG, American College of Obstetricians and Gynecologists; USPSTF, US Preventive Services Task Force.

symptoms seem myriad in nature and disconnected from one another. Sometimes the level of emotion being displayed seems above and beyond, or incongruent with, the symptoms being described. After sorting through the details and attempting to configure a broad picture of what is transpiring, psychosocial concerns are often in the mix. A nonexhaustive list of such concerns includes depression, anxiety, stress (eg, finances, work, relationship dynamics), eating disorders, drug and alcohol abuse and addiction, family discord, marital strife, abuse and trauma history, and grief.

Rather than referring to a mental health department where wait times may be long and assessment practices may delay counseling even further, a same-day consultation or one that can occur in a timely manner, allows the patient to be heard, to engage in problem-solving, and to garner support. The clinician can assess whether brief/time-limited counseling can be done by him/her in the medical department, or if the issues are more complicated and require referral. An important assessment by the women's health psychologist is whether the patient has any indication of a bipolar disorder or a psychotic condition. This information is essential in deciding whether to refer to a psychiatry department and in how patients are counseled for their options around psychotropic medications.

Beyond general emotional health concerns, issues specific to women's health can cause significant levels of distress and reduced quality of life. Examples include coping with premenstrual syndrome/premenstrual dysphoric disorder (PMS/PMDD), handling the changes that accompany perimenopause/menopause, addressing sexual functioning challenges, confronting fertility challenges, pregnancy decision-making (ie, termination, deciding how to proceed and/or cope when fetal complications have been detected, whether to have more children and birth spacing), addressing the emotions that accompany diagnosis and treatment of gynecologic cancers, coping with pelvic pain, and coping after pregnancy loss. Clinical intervention with presenting issues such as these requires knowledge not only of the medical condition, but of the common emotional and psychological sequelae of these experiences. The women's health psychologist is uniquely skilled at bridging the connections between the medical and the psychological and then offering feedback and tools that can help the patient feel understood, empowered to make wellness changes, and cope better.

Tools are available to help primary care physicians get a sense of how patients are psychologically faring with many of these aforementioned conditions. However, knowing that a psychiatric diagnosis or a psychosocial stressor is present does not mean that one has the skill, time, or ability to address the psychological needs of the patient. Regarding detection and management of perinatal depression (ie, antenatal and postpartum), a recent analysis found that 50% to 70% of cases are undetected, 85% are untreated, and 91% to 93% are not adequately treated.[19] This is what the colocated mental health clinician would be able to skillfully weigh-in on and then take on their share of the treatment plan. This model is satisfying to patients and providers.

Brief and time-limited psychotherapeutic interventions would be centered around enhancement of coping skills, review and improvement of communication skills, teaching relational health and recommending behavior-based homework, sharing information about assertiveness, and promoting self-care. A cognitive-behavioral (CB) framework is used to help patients understand the interplay between their thoughts, physiology, emotions, and behaviors. Once this knowledge is established, CB tools are implemented to dissect one's thoughts and behaviors with the intent of ushering in more accurate/balanced thoughts and healthier behaviors. For example, in patients with pelvic pain conditions, such as endometriosis, high rates of depression and anxiety have been found and psychological intervention has been recommended to help with perceptions of pain and to proactively tackle quality-of-life concerns.[20] Furthermore, the European Association of Urology has called for broadening treatment protocols in women with chronic pelvic pain; they encourage treatment to be integrated such that attention is paid to the medical, psychosocial, and sexual aspects of the pain condition.[21]

For behavioral changes to stick and become true lifestyle changes, there must be a commitment to tracking behavior, mindfully setting reasonable goals, delaying gratification, and building in a new set of rewards. Relatedly, the perspective of the embedded medical psychologist allows for continual focus on health promotion. Each session with the patient would include some discussion of health behaviors, such as healthy diet, engagement in regular exercise, smoking cessation, safe sexual practices, routine engagement in pleasurable activities, and stress management. An overarching goal with health promotion is to have the patient understand how much of their wellness is under their control and can be addressed outside of the medical system. Said conversely, most disease burden is caused by lifestyle and behavioral choices that are alterable (**Box 1**).[22]

Preconception

Starting from the beginning of a possible perinatal journey, a psychologist could prove integral when patients present for a preconception visit. As patients sort out their readiness and wellness for pregnancy, many psychosocial factors may come into play. These include personal and familial psychiatric history, lifetime exposure to trauma, relationship health, and basic safety and wellness needs (eg, food security, community safety, stable employment, financial stability, and established social networks where one has regular access to emotional support). Motivational interviewing and introduction of skills to facilitate behavior change may prove enlightening and encouraging to women who hope to emotionally and behaviorally position themselves well before conception. Additionally, some women may require more in-depth psychotherapy to come to terms with the sequelae from past traumas or other long-standing psychiatric symptoms. The mental health clinician would be able to assess the patient's psychological background and current stressors, review current functioning, establish the patient's motivations and goals around having children, and then be able to make suggestions for the course of subsequent treatment.

Prenatal Psychology

Prevalence rates for perinatal mood and anxiety disorders (PMAD) during pregnancy are estimated to be 20% in high-income countries and perhaps even higher in low- to middle-income nations.[23] Certain subpopulations tend to have higher rates of PMAD. These include the impoverished, teenagers, women of color, and women living in violent relationships. Evidence[24] is debunking the long-held belief that pregnancy is

---

Box 1
Psychosocial screening tools

Open Access Screening Tools:
   Depression (PHQ9) and anxiety (GAD7): https://www.phqscreeners.com/select-screener/41
   Social determinants of health: https://www.chcs.org/resource/screening-social-deteiminants-health-populations-complex-needs-implementation-considerations/
   Adverse childhood experiences questionnaire: http://www.ncjfcj.org/sites/default/files/Finding%20Your%20ACE%20Score.pdf
   Domestic and sexual violence questionnaires: https://www.cdc.gov/violenceprevention/pdf/ipv/ipvandsvscreening.pdf
   Female sexual functioning: https://www.aafp.org/afp/2011/0915/p705.html
   https://www.researcheate.net/figure/The-modified-Brief-Sexual-Symptom-Checklist-for-Women-BSSC- W_fig1_277610474
   Post-traumatic stress disorder checklist: http://www.bhevolution.org/public/document/pcl.pdf
   Drug/alcohol screener: http://www.bhevolution.org/public/document/cage-aid.pdf
   Distress among oncology patients: https://www.nccn.org/patients/resources/life with cancer/pdf/nccn distress thermometer.pdf

mood protective and reduces vulnerability to new onset of psychiatric illness or relapse of psychiatric conditions. WPSI recommends screening for depression and intimate partner violence in pregnancy. All women should be screened early in pregnancy for personal and familial history of PMAD and at least one to two more times during pregnancy, along with a postpartum screen. Special attention should be paid to women who are late to enter prenatal care because this can be an indicator of a psychosocial need or distress. It is still common practice for significant numbers of women to discontinue psychotropic use on confirmation of pregnancy status. It is recommended that the medical provider gather information on the pregnant patient's past use of psychotropic drugs, last use of such drugs, and the symptoms since discontinuation of use. A sensitive conversation can then be held about the use of such drugs during pregnancy and/or nursing and what the risks and benefits are to patient and fetus. No psychiatric medication is without risk during pregnancy, and equally importantly, choosing not to medicate a clinically significant psychiatric condition is also not without risk.[25] Impact of maternal psychiatric disturbance has been shown to have significant and broad implications on children's well-being[26] and familial wellness; addressing such concerns proactively is an effective two-generation health intervention.

The psychologist working with pregnant women suffering from PMAD can review the risks of untreated symptoms. These include, but are not limited to, worsening symptoms in the postpartum period; detachment from close friends and family; absenteeism from work; increased desire for cigarettes, drugs, and/or alcohol; dysregulated appetite and sleep patterns; and suicidality. Regardless of whether medication is selected or not by the patient, CB skills can be taught to help with the management of depression and anxiety symptoms. Additionally, a review of social circumstances, relationship needs, and stress management can also be addressed with the pregnant woman by the department psychologist. Addressing these factors in a timely manner may prove empowering to women who want to be well-prepared before birth to handle the new challenges of motherhood.

Subpopulations of women who may require special attention during pregnancy include those who have had a prior history of pregnancy loss, have unplanned pregnancies, have conceived after birth control sabotage, who are now pregnant after experiencing infertility, may not be at peace with their termination histories, and have experienced complications in previous pregnancies and/or deliveries.

Postpartum Conditions

The postpartum period for women is a fragile time marked by significant increase in psychiatric vulnerability and tremendous life change. Sleep is at a minimum, relationships are often taxed, and the focus of care is typically on baby rather than mother. A special issue of the *Journal of Behavioral Medicine* was published in 2018 and called for improved care of women in the fourth trimester.[27,28] The lack of adequate behavioral health care for women was called out and recommendations included expansion of medical teams to include embedded and colocated social workers and health psychologists. Unaddressed maternal psychological distress thwarts the mother/baby bond and puts other preexisting relationships with spouses and older children in jeopardy. Interventions should be patient-centered, available for timely consultation, and delivered through diverse means (eg, telephone, groups, individual counseling, examination room consultation).

The ubiquitous term "postpartum depression" obfuscates the number of women who are suffering from postpartum anxieties, including panic disorder, obsessive-compulsive disorder, and post-traumatic stress disorder. Anxiety conditions are often the comorbid preexisting conditions that accompany perinatal depression. More than 60% of women with perinatal depression had a comorbid psychiatric condition, and of these, more than 80% were anxiety disorders.[29] Other psychological conditions that require postpartum attention include bipolar disorder and psychosis. Wisner and coworkers[29] assert that detection of bipolar disorder is the most important prerequisite for adequate psychiatric treatment. In her population of women who screened positive for postpartum depression, 22% had bipolar disorder. Risk factors for all these diagnoses include personal and familial history of such conditions, the presentation of related symptoms during pregnancy, and challenges during the prenatal period or delivery experience. Strained marital relations, including those that pose danger of violence, and limited social support after bringing baby home can further stress the psychological milieu. The behavioral health professional can work with women affected by PMAD by promoting more balanced expectations of one's self and prescribing self-care (making time to eat, granting permission to shower, tending to activities of daily living, reintroducing exercise when appropriate, and prioritizing sleep [eg, teaching sleep hygiene skills and encouraging use of social supports to increase the time available for sleep]). Therapeutic groups provide normalization and strategies for addressing many of the common concerns raised by postpartum mothers; these include disappointment as a result of unmet birth plans, breastfeeding challenges, experiencing less than adequate support from fathers and other family members, shifts in body image, profound changes in identity and self-perception, concerns about returning to work, and handling the ongoing needs and possible regressions in older children.

In a 2017 meta-analysis done with women who have experienced postpartum depression, themes emerged around access to care and the most salient aspects of care once psychological intervention was accepted.[30] The studies included in the analysis were multinational and what emerged was a hesitancy to seek out psychological care because of stigma, fear of being perceived as a bad mother, and a sense that a fragmented health care system would not be able to offer the right kind of services (ie, mother-focused, sufficiently knowledgeable about postpartum conditions, confidential, and a continuous relationship with a care provider with whom they felt rapport). All of these concerns are much more easily addressed when a psychologist is embedded in an OB/GYN department. This professional can continuously serve as educator to his/her medical peers (eg, MDs, NPs, CNMs, LACs, PharmDs) and create patient-friendly literature and signage that conveys the department's care and skill at addressing peripartum mood concerns. Likewise, the provider focused on caring for pregnant and postpartum women brings to the table the "soft skills" (listening skills, empathy, unconditional regard, nonjudgmental stance) and "hard skills" (ability to incorporate efficacious psychological interventions; knowledge about psychiatric trends and vulnerabilities during the time periods before, during, and after pregnancy; skill to discuss psychotropic medications; and the ability to stay mother- and relationship-focused at a time period when many women believe that the focus is now primarily on their babies) that the peripartum population wants and needs. Universally, women want to believe that they are well enough to be able to be the types of mothers that they wish to be. When motherhood is preceded or met with psychological hurdles it takes clinical skill to help the new mother rebuild her confidence, guide her through appropriate CB skills so that wellness is re-established or inaugurated, and provide psychoeducation to foster self-esteem, assertiveness, effective communication, and healthy relationships (**Table 2**).

Table 2
Prevalence, onset, duration, and treatment for common postpartum psychiatric conditions

Disorder	Prevalence (%)	Onset	Duration	Treatment
Blues	30–75	Postpartum Day 3–4	Hours to days	None, assurance
Postpartum depression	10–15	Within 12 mo	Week to months	Meds, psychotherapy
Postpartum anxiety	10–15			
Postpartum psychosis	0.1–0.2	Typically, within 2 wk of delivery	Weeks to months	Hospitalization

Hormonal Concerns

For many patients, it may be more palatable or ego syntonic to use medical rather than psychological language to describe their symptoms and concerns. OB/GYNs routinely get asked by patients for laboratory studies to be drawn to establish whether hormones are within normal range. Examples of clinical conditions where this may be the case include PMS/PMDD, polycystic ovarian syndrome, infertility, and perimenopause/menopause. As an adjunct to the medical explanations and interventions, the psychologist can add to the patient's treatment plan around such concerns. The impact of all these aforementioned conditions on the patient's relational dynamics should be constructively explored and communication skills can be bolstered so that the patient can understand why she may be experiencing increased emotional dysregulation or volatility. In turn, self-regulation can be worked on, as could effective communication skills, conflict management, self-care, and behavioral goal-setting. The psychologist can explore with the patient what other life forces are simultaneously present that may be exacerbating the behavioral and emotional dysregulation. For example, women going through menopause are often referred to as being the "sandwich generation," and may be in the midst of high-stake caregiving for children and parents. For all the aforementioned conditions, it is helpful to explore what is happening relationally (sources of comfort vs where there is discord) and professionally (demands, support, recognition, satisfaction, work/life balance). Assessing for individual strengths can then guide the recommendations for how to approach hardships and challenges. Comparison with family members, close friends, and peers may contribute to self-attributions that one is failing, falling behind, or inadequate. Women of child-bearing age who are having troubles with conceiving may become despondent or panicky about having a dream unfulfilled or getting left behind by friends who are moving on to the next chapters in their lives. PMS/PMDD, polycystic ovarian syndrome, infertility, and the menopause transition all have the power to evoke negative appraisals around body image. A sense of control is regained when patients are coached to set reasonable and measurable goals around diet and exercise and to use CB skills to effectively alter self-talk and self-assessment. Relatedly, once the patient's personal narrative around her hardship is elicited, it can be dismantled and then reconstructed to a story that is hopefully infused with hope, agency, and purpose.

Relational/Sexual Abuse

Rates of domestic violence are staggering nationally and internationally.[31] WPSI believes that screening for intimate partner violence is an important element of well-woman health care. Violence prevention efforts by public health agencies and health care systems are desperately needed and this should include education around healthy relationships and recovery from lifetime exposure to relational aggression.

Conceptualization of the problem and scope of intervention should include the whole continuum from emotional abuse through physical and sexual abuse/violence. Sometimes patients speak-up without prompting about what they have experienced and what they need for their healing and many more times, we miss these cases when we do not sensitively and directly ask about relational safety and when these boundaries have been transgressed. The embedded mental professional can talk to violence survivors about establishing safety; the impact of violence on one's physical and psychological health; and relatedly, the impact on child witnesses. They can also help establish what psychological sequelae may be present and help direct patients toward federally funded community agencies, which focus specifically on intimate partner violence and sexual assault.

The embedded women's health psychologist could serve as clinic lead in education about domestic violence and lead the efforts around screening and referral. Routine inquiry should always be done about history of physical and sexual abuse and clinical presentations that may accompany such a history include: elevated anxiety with or avoidance of pelvic examinations, concerning/controlling behaviors by accompanying partners to office visits, and explanations for injuries that are not congruous with the presenting complaints or injuries. The medical provider's assurance to patients that they are not to blame for violence that they have sustained and that they are deserving of happiness and safety are effective and invaluable interventions. Even more so, the referral to a trusted mental health colleague shows alliance between words and action (ie, asking about domestic violence and then not only wanting to help with the problem when it has been disclosed, but having readily available resources to refer to) and takes empathy to the level of finding solutions. In solo practice, one way of establishing a relationship with a trusted mental health colleague could be through a colocation agreement or by sharing a mental health practitioner with another solo practice or group of practitioners.

Sexual abuse may present in an OB/GYN department as an acute incident of sexual assault that may be distal or proximal or a trauma that was chronically faced in the patient's life perhaps in childhood or adulthood or both. Sexual violence is an umbrella term that describes any unwanted and nonconsensual sexual behavior that someone may have been exposed to (eg, incest, sexual harassment, forced or coerced touch, trafficking, stalking, exposure to degrading sexual imagery). Approximately 19% of women in the United States have been raped and 44% have been exposed to some form of sexual violence.[32] Childhood survivors of sexual abuse in adulthood are four times more likely to develop drug abuse, four times more likely to suffer from post-traumatic stress disorder, and three times more likely to experience major depression than those without such history.[33] The provider's skill and awareness around being trauma-informed can make a substantial impact on the patient and her subsequent willingness to pursue psychological counseling. Tremendous shame can accompany such a history and the provider's empathic listening and supportive comments could be the patient's first step toward healing and establishment of physical and mental safety.

Adverse Childhood Experiences and Other Trauma History

There is now a burgeoning literature and science on the impact of adverse childhood experiences (ACEs) and health. The movement was started by Drs Felitti (Kaiser Permanente, San Diego) and Anda (Centers for Disease Control and Prevention) and 20 plus years out from their seminal paper,[34] health care systems are still trying to operationalize how best to assess for lifetime exposure to psychosocial trauma, coordinate referrals for care, and structure interventions that enhance resilience while also promoting healing from the sequelae of trauma. ACEs fall into one of three categories: (1) abuse (physical, emotional, sexual), (2) neglect (physical and emotional), and (3) household dysfunction (exposure to parental incarceration, domestic violence, mental illness, substance abuse, and divorce). The original study found that 64% of the study population (n = 17,000+) had at least one ACE and among that group, 87% had two or more ACEs. Having exposure to four or more ACEs (16% of people) is the critical juncture at which significant impact on mental and physical health have been repeatedly found. Examples include significantly higher rates of health risk behaviors (eg, smoking, drug and alcohol abuse, overeating) and overall disease (eg, risk for ischemic heart disease, stroke, and cancer are doubled from those with zero ACEs). For people with six or more ACEs, risk for suicidality goes up 30-fold. The impact of maternal ACEs on birth outcomes and infant/child mental health is also now being studied. A recent study found a strong link between maternal smoking in those with significant history of ACEs and subsequent obstetric outcomes of shortened gestational age and reduced birth weight.[35] Assessing ACEs history along with resilience level (ie, low vs high) can assist in identifying pregnant and postpartum women who would most benefit from psychosocial intervention.[36]

It is often during pregnancy where women present with hope for the future, a desire to undo the harmful experiences of their pasts, and create better lives for their offspring. This offers a unique and critical opportunity for embedded mental health clinicians to reach these women and help unpack the impact of trauma exposure and teach new skills that foster healthy attachment, regulation of emotions, and effective parenting skills (eg, establishment of routines, naming of emotions and responding appropriately, serve and return skills). Results of a small qualitative study found that patients are more willing to engage in behavioral health appointments around psychosocial adversity if the provider was directly embedded in their primary care provider's department.[37] Expectations can be set reasonably when mothers-to-be are given

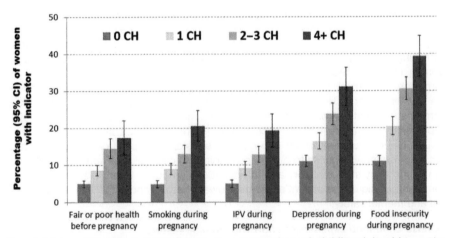

Fig. 1. Maternal health indicators according to number of childhood hardships. The Maternal and Infant Health Assessment is an annual population-based survey of women with a recent live birth with a sample size of n = 13,663 in 2011–2012. Percentages and 95% confidence intervals are weighted to represent all women with a live birth in 2011–2012 in California. CH, childhood hardship; CI, confidence interval. (*Courtesy of* the California Department of Public Health, Maternal, Child and Adolescent Health Division, Sacramento, CA, © (2014) California Department of Public Health.)

information on child developmental and how to respond to the inevitable challenges and frustrations that arise with the care of infants. Most importantly, primary prevention can be initiated in helping parents not replicate intergenerational patterns secondary to trauma and thereby, reduce likelihood of their children ultimately being subjected to ACEs. Powerful interventions that can help achieve this goal include altering relational dysfunction and addressing domestic violence, establishing psychiatric treatment of parental mental illness, and connecting parents with social services that could help meet basic needs. Resilience is nurtured by safe, stable, and nurturing relationships. Health care providers are positioned to model such behavior for their patients. As trust is established in the clinical relationship, the hope is that patients can transfer newly gained skills to their personal lives and thereby reduce transmission of further distress and dysfunction (**Fig. 1**).

SUMMARY

In the OB/GYN arena, patients presenting with psychosocial concerns and distress is common. Comprehensive, efficacious, and meaningful health care requires adequate attention be paid to the physiologic and the psychological symptoms of the patient. Interdisciplinary intervention within the same department, by colleagues who work side by side each day, is the model of the future. The need is there, providers and patients have shown preference for such a structure, and the outcomes are promising.

REFERENCES

1. Hanlon P, Carlisle S, Hannah M, et al. Making the case for a 'fifth wave' in public health. Public Health 2011;125(1):30–6.
2. Preamble to the constitution of the World Health Organization as adopted by the International Health Organization. Available at: http://www.who.int/suggestions/faq/en/.
3. Accortt EE, Wong MS. It is time for routine screening for perinatal mood and anxiety disorders in obstetrics and gynecology settings. Obstet Gynecol Surv 2017; 72(9):553–68.
4. Sacks A. The birth of a mother. The New York Times; 2017. Available at: https://www.nytimes.com/2017/05/08/well/family/the-birth-of-a-mother.html.
5. American Psychological Association. Briefing series on the role of psychology in health care: integrated health care 2014. Available at: https://www.apa.org/health/briefs/integrated-healthcare.pdf.
6. Available at: https://www.youtube.com/watch?v=BbMGIDtCxew.
7. Poleshuck EL, Woods J. Psychologists partnering with obstetricians and gynecologists: meeting the need for patient-centered models of women's health care delivery. Am Psychol 2014;69(4):344–54.
8. Leddy MA, Lawrence H, Schulkin J. Obstetrician-gynecologists and women's mental health: findings of the collaborative ambulatory research network 2005-2009. Obstet Gynecol Surv 2011;66(5):316–23.
9. Smith MV, Shao L, Howell H, et al. Success of mental health referral among pregnant and postpartum women with psychiatric distress. Gen Hosp Psychiatry 2009;31:155–62.
10. Linton MJ, Dieppe P, Medina-Lara A. Review of 99 self-report measures for assessing well-being in adults: exploring dimensions of well-being and developments over time. BMJ Open 2016;6. https://doi.org/10.1136/bmjopen-2015-010641.

11. Rath T, Harter J. The five essential elements of well-being," Workplace, May 4, 2010.

12. Bursztajn H, Barsky AJ. Facilitating patient acceptance of a psychiatric referral. Arch Intern Med 1985;145:73–5.

13. Available at: http://www.psychiatrictimes.com/major-depressive-disorder/helping-primary-care-physicians-make-psychiatric-referrals.

14. Byatt N, Levin LL, Ziedonis D, et al. Enhancing participation in depression care in outpatient perinatal care settings: a systematic review. Obstet Gynecol 2015; 126(5):1048–58.

15. Maslow AH. Motivation and personality. Oxford (England): Harpers; 1954

16. Available at: https://www.211ca.org/.

17. Available at: https://www.cdc.gov/socialdeterminants/.

18. Cole HE, Rojas PX, Joseph J. Building a movement to birth a more just and loving world. National Perinatal Task Force 2018. Available at: https://drive.google.com/file/d/0B_vxE9qdE1jDZ2Q2TGpLaTB6ME1qSGgyeDFkYnd5b0dRSWxV/view.

19. Cox EQ, Sowa NA, Meltzer-Brody SE, et al. The perinatal depression treatment cascade: baby steps toward improving outcomes. J Clin Psychiatry 2016; 77(9):1189–200.

20. Lagana AS, LaRosa LV, Rapisarda AMC, et al. Anxiety and depression in patients with endometriosis: impact and management challenges. Int J Womens Health 2017;9:323–30.

21. Engeler DS, Baranowski AP, Dinis-Oliveira P, et al. The 2013 EAU guidelines on chronic pelvic pain: is management of chronic pelvic pain a habit, a philosophy, or a science? 10 years of development. Eur Urol 2013;64(3):431–9.

22. Institute of Medicine. Health and behavior: the interplay of biological, behavioral, and societal influences. Washington, DC: The National Academies Press; 2001.

23. Biaggi A, Conroy S, Pawlby S, et al. Identifying the women at risk of antenatal anxiety and depression: a systematic review. J Affect Disord 2016;191:62–77.

24. Cohen LS, Nonacs RM, Bailey JW, et al. Relapse of depression during pregnancy following antidepressant discontinuation: a preliminary prospective study. Arch Womens Ment Health 2004;7(4):217–21.

25. Chisholm MS, Payne JL. Management of psychotropic drugs during pregnancy. BMJ 2015;351:1–15.

26. Glover V. Maternal depression, anxiety and stress during pregnancy and child outcome; what needs to be done. Best Pract Res Clin Obstet Gynaecol 2014; 28:25–35.

27. Hamilton N, Stevens N, Lillis T, et al. The fourth trimester: toward improved postpartum health and healthcare of mothers and their families in the United States. J Behav Med 2018;41(5):571–6.

28. Verbiest S, Tully K, Simpson M, et al. Elevating mothers' voices: recommendations for improved patient-centered postpartum. J Behav Med 2018;41(5): 577–90.

29. Wisner KL, Sit DKY, McShea MC, et al. Onset timing, thoughts of self-harm, and diagnoses in postpartum women with screen-positive depression findings. JAMA Psychiatry 2013;70(5):490–8.

30. Hadfield H, Wittkowski A. Women's experiences of seeking and receiving psychological and psychosocial interventions for postpartum depression: a systematic review and thematic synthesis of the qualitative literature. J Midwifery Womens Health 2017;62(6):723–36.

31. Garcia-Moreno C, Jansen HAFM, Ellsberg M, et al. Prevalence of intimate partner violence: findings from the WHO multi-country study on women's health and domestic violence. Lancet 2006;368(9551):1937.
32. Breiding MJ, Smith SG, Basile KC, et al. Prevalence and characteristics of sexual violence, stalking, and intimate partner violence victimization – National intimate partner and sexual violence survey, United States, 2011. MMWR Surveill Summ 2014;63(8):1–18.
33. Available at: https://www.rainn.org/statistics/children-and-teens.
34. Felitti VJ, Anda RA, Nordenberg D, et al. Relationship of childhood abuse and household dysfunction to many of the leading causes of death in adults. Am J Prev Med 1998;14(4):245–58.
35. Smith MV, Gotman N, Yonkers KA. Early childhood adversity and pregnancy outcomes. Matern Child Health J 2016;20(4):790–8.
36. Young-Wolff KC, Alabaster A, McCaw B, et al. Adverse childhood experiences and mental and behavioral health conditions during pregnancy: the role of resilience. J Womens Health 2018;00(00):1–10.
37. Vu C, Rothman E, Kistin CJ, et al. Adapting the patient-centered medical home to address psychosocial adversity: results of a qualitative study. Acad Pediatr 2017; 17(7S):S115–22.

Cancer Screening in Women

Alison Vogell, MD*, Megan L. Evans, MD, MPH

KEYWORDS

- Female cancer screening • Female cancer statistics • Cancer screening guidelines

KEY POINTS

- Cancer screening is of paramount importance to reduce early morbidity and mortality in women.
- Screening modalities should balance risks of delaying cancer diagnosis against harms of over-testing and over-diagnosis.
- Timing and frequency of screening can vary and should be based on a shared decision model between the patient and her physician.
- Patients at increased risk of certain types of cancer may benefit from earlier and more frequent screening strategies.
- Clinicians should identify nonmodifiable risk factors in patients and counsel regarding lifestyle modifications where feasible.

INTRODUCTION

The Women's Preventive Services Initiative (WPSI) aims to improve women's health across the life span and to complement, build on, and fill gaps in existing guidelines provided by the United States Preventive Services Task Force (USPSTF). This goal is particularly important around cancer screening, where differing recommendations may be made by each society. The authors summarize WPSI in each section and review key recommendations from relevant societies based on each type of cancer for which there are current screening guidelines. Personalized strategies should be designed with both patient and physician input and with the flexibility to accommodate a shared decision-making model. Although these guidelines are validated by data and influenced by expert opinions in their respective fields, they are effective only when a patient herself ascribes value to the recommendation, making it her own health care priority.

Breast Cancer

Among all cancers, breast cancer remains the most commonly diagnosed cancer among women. In 2018, there were an estimated 268,600 new cases of breast cancer

Disclosure Statement: The authors have nothing to disclose.
Department of Obstetrics and Gynecology # 22, Tufts Medical Center, 800 Washington Street, Boston, MA 02111, USA
* Corresponding author.
E-mail address: avogell@tuftsmedicalcenter.org

Obstet Gynecol Clin N Am 46 (2019) 485–499
https://doi.org/10.1016/j.ogc.2019.04.007
0889-8545/19/© 2019 Elsevier Inc. All rights reserved.

obgyn.theclinics.com

and 41,760 associated deaths.[1] The most recent data suggest that 1 in 8 women will be diagnosed with breast cancer in her lifetime, with overall incidence rates increasing slightly by 0.4% per year. In general, mortality rates have declined since peaking in 1989, at 33.2 per 100,000. In 2016, they had decreased by 40% to a rate of 20 deaths per 100,000 women.[1] Improved mortality statistics are likely due to improvements in early detection as well as general awareness of breast health and signs and symptoms of concerning changes in a woman's breast. Despite this overall improvement, rates for black women have increased, highlighting ongoing disparities in access to care.[1]

A major goal of WPSI is to create a consensus for breast cancer screening because women receive different recommendations, depending on the source of the recommendation. As a collaboration of medical organizations and based on scientific evidence, WPSI provides direction on screening across the life span. WPSI recommends that women should initiate screening mammography no earlier than age 40 and no later than age 50 for women at average risk for breast cancer. Screening should continue through at least age 74 and age alone should not be the basis to discontinue screening.

Screening Guidelines

Clinical breast examination

Clinical breast examination (CBE) recommendations vary regarding intervals in asymptomatic average-risk women. Although they are routinely done, there are often higher rates of false positive with perceived abnormal findings noted in the clinic. It has been estimated that for every 1 case of cancer detected after an initial CBE, there were 55 false-positive tests that occurred.[2]

These are the current recommendations for CBE by expert panels and professional societies:

- American Cancer Society (ACS) does not recommend routine CBE.
- USPST does not recommend for or against CBE.
- American College of Obstetricians and Gynecologists (ACOG) recommends offering every 1 year to 3 years for women 25 years to 39 year old and yearly for women 40 and older.
- National Comprehensive Cancer Network (NCCN) has the same recommendation as ACOG.

Additionally, encouraging women to perform self-breast examinations is controversial and can lead to increased false-positive testing. Alternatively, women should be encouraged to engage in breast self-awareness. This empowers women to recognize changes to their breast, including composition, nipple discharge, or drainage or any new masses or lumps. More than half of women detected their own breast cancer while engaging in breast self-awareness.[3]

Mammogram screening

Current recommendations from expert panels and professional societies:

- ACS recommends starting screening at age 45 but can offer initiation of mammograms starting at age 40. Women can be screened biennially, then considering annually starting at age 55. Women may consider stopping when life expectancy is less than 10 years.
- USPTF recommend initiating mammography at age 50. Screening between ages 40 and 49 should be a discussion between a patient and her physician in which risks and benefits can be discussed. Once mammograms are started, they should be done every other year. USPTF states there is not enough evidence to adequately determine the age of stopping breast cancer screening.

- ACOG believes mammography should be started at age 40 or starting in a woman's 40s. Mammography can be continued yearly or biennially and continued until age 75. Decision to continue after age 75 should be a shared decision-making model by a patient and her physician.
- NCCN recommends starting annual screening at age 40 and discontinuing screening when life expectancy is less than 10 years.

There are pros and cons to earlier screening and more frequent testing. Although shorter interval testing can have earlier detection rates and improved health outcomes, it also can lead to increased callback and unnecessary invasive testing. A review from the Breast Cancer Surveillance Consortium found a 10-year cumulative false-positive rate of 42% with biennial screening but a 61% false-positive rate with annual screening. The USPTF found women who had annual screening starting at age 40 had 1 fewer cancer death (8 vs 7), 152 life years versus 122 life years gained, higher false-positive rates, higher episodes of unnecessary breast biopsies, and 21 versus 19 over-diagnosed breast tumors compared with women who had biennial screening starting at age 50.[4] Additionally, women who are called back for false-positive testing may be responsible for the additional cost, can have increased anxiety and stress, and may be less likely to return for future testing. WPSI encourages using this information to inform shared decision making between a woman and her health care provider.

Increased screening also can lead to increased radiation exposure. Women who are screening annually starting at age 40 may result in 11 per 100,000 radiation-induced cancers compared with 2 per 100,000 in women ages 50 to 59 who participate in biennial screening.[4]

Special Populations

There are some populations that have increased risk of breast cancer given past treatment and breast characteristics:

- Young women treated for Hodgkin lymphoma with therapeutic chest radiation have an overall increased risk of breast cancer. This is particularly true for young girls treated between ages 10 and 14.[5]
- Women with dense breasts in Breast Imaging Reporting and Data System categories 3 and 4 have a 1.2 and 2.1 respectively relative risk of breast cancer compared with women with average breast density.[6]
- Women in whom atypical ductal or lobular hyperplasia and lobular carcinoma in situ were found incidentally have a 4-fold risk of invasive cancer in either the same breast and possible the contralateral breast.[7]
- Women exposed to diethylstilbestrol as a fetus carry an almost 2-fold risk of breast cancer.[8]

Screening for patients with genetic mutations

Models like BRCAPRO can help clinicians assess if their patients would benefit from genetic testing for genetic mutations associated with breast and ovarian cancer, specifically BRCA mutation.

Patients who are BRCA positive should have earlier or more frequent breast cancer screening given their increase rates of breast cancer, ranging from 45% to 85% by age 70[9]:

- Women ages 25 to 29 should have CBEs every 6 months to 12 months and annual imaging, preferable MRI with contrast.

- Women ages 30 and above should have annual mammography and annual MRI, alternating every 6 months, as well as yearly CBEs.
- Bilateral mastectomy also should be discussed with the patients because this can decrease their rate of breast cancer by 85% to 100%.

Risk Factors and Prevention

The main risk factor for breast cancer remains the female gender. More than 99% of breast cancers occur in women. Additionally, breast cancer risk increases with age. In general, women who have been diagnosed with invasive breast cancer do not have specific risk factors or common features (**Box 1**).

Breast cancer risk assessment should be performed on every patient to determine timing of screening. This may include risk factors, discussed previously, as well as personal or family history of germline mutation–associated cancers. These may include breast, ovarian, prostate, colon, and/or pancreatic cancer. Risk assessment tools can be used to determine an individual's lifetime risk of breast cancer. These tools can include Gail model, BRCAPRO, Breast and Ovarian Analysis of Disease Incidence and Carrier Estimation Algorithm, and other models.

These tools can help determine if a woman would benefit from genetic testing; enhanced screening, such as MRI; specific risk reduction strategies; and/or CBE.

Box 1
Breast cancer risk factors

- Family history of breast cancer, ovarian cancer, or other hereditary breast and ovarian syndrome–associated cancer (eg, prostate cancer or pancreatic cancer)
- Known deleterious gene mutation
- Prior breast biopsy with specific pathology
  ○ Atypical hyperplasia (lobular or ductal)
  ○ Lobular carcinoma in situ
- Early menarche
- Late menopause
- Nulliparity
- Prolonged interval between menarche and first pregnancy
- Menopausal hormone therapy with estrogen and progestin (decreased risk with estrogen alone)
- Not breastfeeding
- Increasing age
- Certain ethnicities (eg, increased risk of BRCA mutation in Ashkenazi Jewish women)
- Higher body mass index
- Alcohol consumption
- Smoking
- Dense breasts on mammography
- Prior exposure to high-dose therapeutic chest irradiation in young women (10–30 years old)

Reprinted with permission from Breast cancer risk assessment and screening in average-risk women. Practice Bulletin No. 179. American College of Obstetricians and Gynecologists. Obstet Gynecol 2017;130:e1–16.

Cervical Cancer

Cervical cancer incidence has dramatically declined since the introduction of the Pap smear in the early 1940s. Prior to this time, cervical cancer was one of the leading causes of cancer death among women in the United States.[10] From 1975 to 2011, a greater than 50% reduction in cervical cancer rate and mortality occurred.[11] Today, in the United States, more than 12,000 new cases of cervical cancer are projected to be diagnosed in 2019, and more than 4000 women are expected to succumb to the disease on an annual basis.[1] Continued diligence by primary care clinicians to ensure adherence to current screening guidelines remains of paramount importance because most new cases of cancer are largely to be believed in patients who did not receive adequate screening.

The WPSI recommends cervical cancer screening for average-risk women ages 21 years to 65 years. For women ages 21 years to 29 years, the WPSI recommends cervical cancer screening using cervical cytology (Pap smear) every 3 years. Cotesting with cytology and human papillomavirus testing is not recommended for women younger than 30 years. Women ages 30 years to 65 years should be screened with cytology and human papillomavirus testing every 5 years or cytology alone every 3 years. Women who are at average risk should not be screened more than once every 3 years.

Screening Guidelines

Nearly all cases of cervical cancer are caused by high-risk human papillomavirus (hrHPV). Current guidelines have been updated several times in the past few decades to incorporate both cervical cytology and testing for hrHPV. Use of each test varies according to patient age and certain high-risk features. Options for screening include

- Cytology alone testing
- hrHPV testing alone
- hrHPV plus cytology (cotest)

The most recent screening guidelines endorsed by ACOG incorporate recommendations made by the ACS, the American Society for Colposcopy and Cervical Pathology (ASCCP), and the American Society for Clinical Pathology.[12] Updates to further incorporate the use of hrHPV screening were made by the ASCCP and Society of Gynecologic Oncology in 2015.[13] More recently, the USPSTF in 2018 finalized their cervical cancer screening recommendations, endorsing hrHPV screening alone as a strategy for screening women ages 30 to 65.[14]

The most recent guidelines for cervical cancer screening in average-risk patients are summarized in **Table 1**.

The following screening intervals are intended to allow for a balance between high likelihood of cancer detection with minimization of the burdens of screening.

For patients at average risk of cervical cancer, the following guidelines apply[11,14]:

- Screening should begin at age 21.
  - The age at which a patient initiates sexual intercourse or other behavioral factors does not have an impact on the age at which screening should begin.
- Women between ages 21 and 29 should be screened with cytologic testing alone every 3 years.
  - Reflex testing for HPV is performed in the setting of abnormal cytology results.
- Women between ages 30 and 65 may choose either cotesting every 5 years, cytology alone every 3 years, or hrHPV testing alone.
  - Cotesting is the preferred method of testing according to ACOG.
  - The USPSTF endorses all 3 methods as equivalent options, recommending hrHPV testing alone every 5 years.

Table 1
Screening strategies for cervical cancer in patients at average risk

	Cytology Alone	Cytology + High-risk Human Papillomavirus	High-risk Human Papillomavirus Alone
Age <21	None	None	None
Ages 21–29	Every 3 y	None	Every 3 y at ages 25–65[13]
Ages 30–65	Every 3 y	Every 5 y	Every 5 y[14]
Age >65	None[a]	None[a]	None[a]

[a] Patient must have had adequate negative screening in prior 10 years with most recent screening being within the past 5 years.
Adapted from Committee on Practice Bulletins – Gynecology. Practice Bulletin No. 168: Cervical cancer screening and prevention. Obstet Gynecol 2016;128(4):e111–30; and Saslow D, Solomon D, Lawson HW, et al. American Cancer Society, American Society for Colposcopy and Cervical Pathology, and American Society for Clinical Pathology screening guidelines for the prevention and early detection of cervical cancer. CA Cancer J Clin 2012;62(3):147–72; with permission.

- o There is currently only 1 validated, Food and Drug Administration (FDA)-approved test for performing primary hrHPV testing.
- Screening may be discontinued in women after age 65.
  - o Screening may be discontinued only after ensuring 10 years of adequate, negative screening has been completed AND ensuring that the most recent Pap smear was within the prior 5 years.
  - o This recommendation is not to be altered when women report a new sexual partner even after age 65.

HPV vaccination status does not change screening guidelines.
Screening for patients in special populations is outlined in **Table 2**.

Table 2
Screening strategies for cervical cancer in special populations patients at increased risk for cervical cancer

	Screening Strategy
History of high-grade dysplasia (CIN 2 or greater, adenocarcinoma in situ)	Screening should continue for 20 y after treatment or regression of the disease following standard screening guidelines[11]
HIV/immunocompromise	Screening should start at whichever of the following comes first: • Age 21 • Within 1 y of diagnosis of HIV in sexually active patient • Within 1 y of onset of sexual activity in HIV-infected patient Screen annually for 3 y after initiation of screening After 3 y extend screening to every 3 y with • Cytology ages 21–30 • Cotesting or cytology alone There is no age at which it is recommended to stop screening[15]
Diethylstilbestrol exposure	Annual screening with cytology[11]

Special Populations

Screening strategies are modified in these populations due to increased risk of developing cervical cancer in their lifetime and include the following:[11,15]

- For women with a history of high-grade dysplasia (cervical intraepithelial neoplasia [CIN] 2 or CIN 3) or prior diagnosis of adenocarcinoma in situ, screening should continue for 20 years after either treatment or spontaneous regression.
  - This may extend the time of screening beyond age 65.
- For women with a diagnosis of HIV, screening intervals are shortened.
  - Cervical cancer screening may be initiated prior to age 21 in 2 circumstances in this population: within 1 year of the onset of sexual activity in those already diagnosed with HIV or, if the woman is already sexually active, within 1 year of new diagnosis of HIV.
  - After initiation of screening, women with HIV should have annual HPV screening for 3 consecutive years. If all tests are negative, the screening interval can be extended to every 3 years.
  - In patients less than age 30 with HIV, screening should be by cytology alone testing.
  - In patients older than 30, screening may include either cotesting or cytology alone.
  - Screening should continue throughout a woman's life and should not be stopped at age 65.
- For women who are immunocompromised for reasons other than HIV, ACOG supports annual cytologic testing but also notes that those guidelines used for HIV-infected patients are also a reasonable alternative.
- For women exposed to diethylstilbestrol in utero, annual cytology should be obtained.
  - Cytology is obtained both from the cervix and from the upper third of the vagina. It is not known at what age this screening should conclude.

Screening recommendations for patients who have undergone prior hysterectomy change according to a patient's history of cervical disease and type of surgery:[11]

- Women who have undergone a total hysterectomy, meaning complete removal of the cervix, and have never had cervical dysplasia should discontinue screening at the time of their surgery.
  - Screening should not be restarted for any reason in these patients regardless of new possible exposure to HPV or changes in a patient's immunocompetence.
- Patients with a history of CIN 2 or greater should continue screening for 20 years after resolution of the dysplastic lesion.
  - ACOG currently supports the use of cytology alone every 3 years in this group and notes that the role of hrHPV testing is not well established. Cytology should be obtained from the vaginal cuff.
- For patients who have had a supracervical hysterectomy and still retain cervical tissue, standard screening protocols should be continued.

Screening strategies for women who have received the HPV vaccination are the same as for those patients who have not received the vaccine.[11]

Risk Factors and Prevention

It should be discussed with patients that most sexually active individuals are exposed to at least 1 type of HPV throughout their lives. Safe sex practices, including consistent use of condoms, communication with partners about history of disease, and appropriate cleaning of sex toys, should be discussed.

Strategies for prevention of cervical cancer should focus on[11]

- Adherence to screening guidelines
- Administration of the HPV vaccine
- Elimination of high-risk behaviors that are associated with more advanced disease
  - Screening for HIV should be performed in accordance with guidelines because patients with HIV are at increased risk of cervical cancer from HPV infection.
  - The effect of tobacco on cervical disease should be addressed with patients and efforts made to counsel and assist patients in smoking cessation.

There have been several iterations of the FDA-approved HPV vaccine, the most recent of which is a 9-valent vaccine that includes protection against 7 hrHPV types and 2 low-risk types that cause condyloma. The vaccine is highly efficacious in preventing HPV related disease. The vaccine should be initiated in both girls and boys at ages 11 to 12.[16] Recently, the FDA approved use of the HPV vaccine up through age 45.[17] Unfortunately, in the United States, widespread use of the vaccine has been unacceptably slow in implementation. It is crucial that health care providers stress the importance of obtaining the vaccine in all eligible patients and specifically address the vaccine's overall safety and efficacy.

Colorectal Cancer

The ACS estimates that in 2019 there will be 49,730 new colorectal cancer diagnoses and the total number of deaths due to the disease will amount to 23,380.[1] Colorectal cancer represents the third most common cause of cancer death in women. Although the overall incidence of colorectal cancer has been down-trending, CRC incidence in patients younger than age 50 actually has been increasing. Younger patients are victims of more aggressive disease at diagnosis. The reasons for this trend are unclear.[18] Today, colorectal cancer is highly preventable and treatable. Current screening modalities allow for accurate diagnosis at early stages of disease, allowing for high survival rates when the disease is identified early on.[19] Similar to cervical cancer, premalignant disease generally is asymptomatic but can be detected as lesions in the colon, which can be removed. If cancer is detected during screening, it often may be identified at an early enough stage of disease to allow for complete resection.[19]

The WPSI recommends screening for colorectal cancer from ages 50 through 75, following the recommendations of the USPSTF.

Screening Guidelines

Because screening programs have been put into effect since the 1970s, the overall rate of death from the disease has decreased markedly and also has allowed for a shift to earlier stage at diagnosis. Changes in risk factor exposure and treatment strategies also have contributed to reduction in overall mortality.[20]

There are several options for screening average-risk patients. Shared decision making should be used when deciding the best method for the patient. What is of utmost importance is that patients are compliant with whichever screening method they choose and demonstrate willingness to repeat this method in the future. Historically, in-office testing was performed during a digital rectal examination using guaiac-based fecal occult blood testing. This method of testing is not acceptable for colorectal screening.[19]

Current options for screening include[19]

- Guaiac-based fecal occult blood testing (requires home collection of multiple samples)
- Fecal immunochemical testing (FIT) (requires home collection of multiple samples)
- Flexible sigmoidoscopy
- Sigmoidoscopy plus FIT
- Colonoscopy
- Stool DNA testing
- CT colonography
- Capsule colonoscopy

Several organizations had developed screening guidelines for colorectal cancer. The most recent guidelines consider evidence regarding efficacy and safety of screening strategies; currently, the USPSTF recommends the following:

- For women between ages 50 and 75, colorectal screening should be performed by fecal occult blood testing, sigmoidoscopy or colonoscopy.[21] The Multi-Society Task Force of Colorectal Cancer (MSTF), which includes the American College of Gastroenterology, the American Gastroenterological Association, and the American Society for Gastrointestinal Endoscopy, issued guidelines in 2017. This group ranked tests according to tiers with higher tier tests representing the strongest recommendations.[22]
- First tier
  - Colonoscopy every 10 years
  - FIT testing annually in those who decline colonoscopy
- Second tier
  - CT colonography every 5 years
  - FIT-fecal DNA test every 3 years
  - Flexible sigmoidoscopy every 5 years to 10 years
- Third tier
  - Capsule colonography is tier 3

The MSTF also has made additional recommendations for special populations[22]:

- African American populations should initiate screening at age 45.
- Individuals should undergo screening every 10 years starting at age 40 who have
  - First-degree relative with colorectal cancer diagnosed later than age 60
  - First-degree relative with an advanced adenoma diagnosed later than age 60
- Individuals should undergo screening every 5 years and start 10 years prior to the age at diagnosis of the youngest affected family member or age 40 in the following circumstances:
  - Family history of colorectal cancer
  - Advanced adenoma in a first-degree relative who is less than 60 years of age
  - Advanced adenoma in 2 first-degree relatives at any age are recommended to undergo screening by colonoscopy every 5 years, beginning 10 years before the age at diagnosis of the youngest affected relative or age 40, whichever is earlier.

According to the MSTF, screening may be discontinued if a patient has prior history of negative screening and has reached age 75 or has a life expectancy of less than 10 years. If patients do not have a history of adequate screening, then they may consider screening up to age 85 based on life expectancy.[22]

In 2018 the ACS published its recommendations for colorectal cancer screening, which largely agreed with those stated by the MSTF. Similarly, individuals are encouraged to perform screening up to age 75 with care individualized for those between ages 76 and 85. One important difference, however, was that the ACS made a "qualified recommendation" that individuals initiate screening at age 45. This group cites recent data that colorectal cancer is being identified in younger populations. The ACS also notes that several tests are appropriate for screening and that, most importantly, the test is acceptable to the patient.[20]

Appropriate screening according to the ACS includes the following[20]:

- FIT annually; high-sensitivity
- Guaiac-based fecal occult blood test annually
- Multitarget stool DNA test every 3 years
- Colonoscopy every 10 years
- CT colonography every 5 years
- Flexible sigmoidoscopy every 5 years

Any positive screening test should be followed-up with a diagnostic procedure, namely colonoscopy.[20,22]

Risk Factors and Prevention

The following circumstances represent women who are of increased risk of colorectal cancer and may be subject to alteration in guidelines and or earlier screening onset[19]:

- Personal history of colorectal polyps or cancer
- Family history of colorectal polyps or cancer
- Personal history of inflammatory bowel disease
- Genetic conditions that predispose women to colorectal cancer, such as hereditary nonpolyposis colorectal cancer syndrome and familial adenomatous polyposis
- History of abdominal radiation
- History of cystic fibrosis

There is an increased risk of colorectal cancer in African Americans.[20]

Lifestyle modifications that may allow for reduction in risk include tobacco cessation, reductions in alcohol use, and eating a healthy diet that is low in red and processed meats and high in fiber, calcium, fruits, and vegetables. Maintaining a healthy weight both through diet and regular exercise can reduce the risk of colorectal cancer as well. The use of aspirin, nonsteroidal anti-inflammatory drugs, and hormone replacement therapy in women may be protective.[22]

Lung Cancer

In the United States, the number 1 cause of cancer death among women is lung cancer. For 2019, the ACS estimates that the number of new lung cancer diagnoses in women will be 111,710 and the number of deaths will amount to 66,020.[1] The most common cause of lung cancer is cigarette smoking and exposure may be either directly through personal use of tobacco or by way of second-hand smoke.[23] The most important way for providers to help their patients prevent lung cancer is with smoking cessation counseling and support.

The WPSI recommends screening for lung cancer in the high-risk population. In other words, women with a 30-pack-year smoking history or women who have quit within the past 15 years should be evaluated.

Screening Guidelines

Initial studies to evaluate lung cancer screening considered the use of chest radiography, sputum cytology, and/or other biological markers. Unfortunately, findings did not support screening by any method because lung cancer mortality was not found reduced in the intervention groups. In 2011, the National Lung Screening Trial, a prospective randomized controlled trial, published findings demonstrating that high-risk patients who were screened with low-dose CT (LDCT) experienced an overall reduction in lung cancer mortality compared with patients being screened with chest radiograph. This trial included both men and women.[24] Several organizations then adapted findings from this trial to create guidelines for lung cancer screening.

The most recently USPSTF guideline for lung cancer screening recommends annual screening with low-dose CT in patients ages 55 to 80 who currently smoke and have a 30-pack-year smoking history or who have quit within the past 15 years.[23]

More recent guidelines published by the American College of Chest Physicians in 2018 evaluate current evidence and highlight the importance of understanding the balance between benefit and harm in widespread adoption of annual LDCT in any population. Specifically, this group highlights weaknesses in evidence supporting which patients should be screened, disparities in imaging between different facilities, and that differences in smoking cessation interventions may affect the quality of LDCT screening. Although annual screening in high-risk patients continues to be supported in these guidelines, this recommendation was noted to be weak. Further recommendations specify that other groups that may be considered high risk based on risk predictor calculators not receive LDCT.[25]

USPSTF is currently updating their 2013 guidelines and a draft summary is available online but not yet finalized at the time of this publication.[26]

Risk Factors and Prevention

Cigarette smoking is the major cause of lung cancer. This risk from smoking increases as the cumulative exposure to cigarette smoke increases. Increasing age is the second most important risk factor. Other less common risk factors include exposure to radon; family history; certain occupational exposures, such as asbestos or arsenic; history of chronic obstructive lung disease; and pulmonary fibrosis.[23]

Risk reduction strategies should include counseling current smokers on cessation as well as advising nonsmokers on how to avoid exposure. Smoking cessation reduces the risk of lung cancer and the overall benefit continues to increase the longer the patient does not smoke. Counseling regarding smoking cessation strategies should include behavioral change and FDA-approved pharmacotherapy options when appropriate.[27]

Ovarian Cancer

Ovarian cancer is the deadliest cancer of the female reproductive system; it ranks fifth for all causes of cancer deaths among women because most women are diagnosed with advanced disease.[1] In 2018, there were 22,240 new cases of ovarian cancers in the United States and just over 14,000 deaths from the disease.[1] A woman's lifetime risk of being diagnosed with ovarian cancer is 1 in 78 whereas the chance of dying from the disease is 1 in 108. The probability of developing ovarian cancer increases with age, peaking at 1 in 265 at age 70 years, with the median age of diagnosis at 63 years. Non-Hispanic white women have a higher incidence of ovarian cancer at 12 per 100,000 women compared with 11.4 per 100,000 for all women and mortality rate at 7.9 per 100,000 women compared with 7 per 100,000 women of all women.

Although black women have a lower incidence rate, at 9.2 per 100,000 women, they have the third highest mortality rate, at 6.1 per 100,000 women just behind American Indian and Alaskan Native women, at 6.3 per 100,000 women.[28] This high mortality rate may be secondary to advanced stage at diagnosis, comorbidities, and lack of access to care.

The WPSI does not recommend screening for ovarian cancer in women of average risk.

Screening Guidelines

Currently there are no screening recommendations for average-risk women. Transvaginal ultrasounds, cancer antigen (CA)-125 serum screening, and bimanual examinations have not been shown to reduce mortality in average-risk women.[29] Results from several studies show false-positive results may lead to unnecessary surgeries and interventions. A study through the United Kingdom Collaborative Trial of Ovarian Cancer screening showed that for every 1 woman diagnosed with ovarian cancer, 10 women had unnecessary surgery based on findings from their imaging.[29] Additionally, using CA-125 alone or other serum testing to assess ovarian cancer risk has not decreased mortality.

Average-risk women who develop concerning symptoms, including bloating, early satiety, and pelvic or abdominal pain, may warrant further evaluation to rule out ovarian cancer. Testing may include a transvaginal ultrasound and/or serum testing.

High-risk Populations

Women who are at high risk of developing ovarian cancer, specifically women with the BRCA mutation, Lynch syndrome, or other genetic mutations, or who have a personal or family history of ovarian cancer may benefit from specific screening tests for ovarian cancer.

Prior to age 30, it is not recommended women undergo routine transvaginal ultrasounds or serum CA-125 levels. Starting at ages 30 to 35, high-risk women may undergo transvaginal screening or CA-125 serum screening per ACOG to assess for risk of ovarian cancer.[30] Alternatively, NCCN recommends women starting at ages 30 to 35 undergo transvaginal ultrasound and CA-125 screening every 6 months.[31]

Risk reducing bilateral salpingo-oophorectomy is encouraged after a woman is done childbearing or at least by age 40. This can reduce the rates of ovarian cancer by 80% and reduce rates of breast cancer in BRCA-positive patients.[30]

Risk Factors and Prevention

Women with a prior history of breast cancer have a nearly 30% risk of developing ovarian cancer in their lifetimes. This is higher if they were diagnosed with breast cancer prior to age 40. This early diagnosis may be associated with gene mutations like BRCA and Lynch syndrome, and screening for ovarian cancer in these patients is discussed later. History of endometriosis, pelvic inflammatory disease, and polycystic ovarian syndrome has been proposed as risk factors for ovarian cancer but their association is uncertain.

There are other exposures and factors that have been shown to both increase and decrease ovarian cancer incidence[1]:

Increase
- Smoking: cigarette smoking has been shown to increase risk, specifically of mucinous ovarian cancer, up to 80%. Overall relative risk is 1.8.

- Postmenopausal hormones: any exposure increased risk to 1.2 in a woman's lifetime. Risk is 40% higher among women who were current or used hormone replacement therapy within 5 years. Most common ovarian cancer types in this population were serous and endometrioid carcinoma (see Mary Jane Minkin's article, "Menopause: Hormones, Lifestyle, and Optimizing Aging," in this issue).
- Obesity: in general, obesity increased risk of epithelial ovarian cancer by 1.1. Obese women who have used hormone replacement therapy increase their risk by 10% for every 5 kg/m^2 of body mass index.
- Exposure to talcum powder: it is unclear if exposure to talcum powder increases risk of ovarian cancer because many studies have had mixed results. Some consumer available talcum powders may contain asbestos, which the International Agency for Research on Cancer has listed as a carcinogen. Currently, there are voluntary guidelines that cosmetic products should be free of detectable levels of asbestos.[32]
- Height: height has been shown to increase risk of ovarian cancer by 1.1 This risk increased by 7% for every 5 cm (cm) above 155 cm (5 feet).

Decrease

- Pregnancy: overall relative risk is reduced to 0.7 with history of pregnancy. After first pregnancy, risk of ovarian cancer is reduced by 40% and 14% for each additional pregnancy. Reduction may be specific to endometrioid and clear cell carcinoma.
- Surgical sterilization: tubal ligation or occlusion can reduce risk of ovarian cancer by 30% whereas complete removal of the fallopian tubes can reduce ovarian cancer risk by 60%. This accounts for an overall risk reduction of 0.7.
- Hormonal birth control: women who used combined hormonal contraception for 5 years to 9 years reduced their risk of ovarian cancer by 35% for an overall relative risk reduction of 0.6. This protective effect is believed to continue up to 10 years after discontinuation of the birth control pills.

SUMMARY

Cancer screening is imperative to identifying a disease before symptoms develop, enabling detection at an early stage and leading to improved health outcomes. Routine screening allows clinicians to work to prevent cancer in their patients as well as treat or prevent precancerous conditions. Access to health care is critical to ensuring women can access timely screening and early prevention of cancers, specifically the ones discussed previously. Further research is needed in all forms of cancer to identify the most effective screening for all demographics. Although insurance access has improved for all women, there is still work to be done to close the disparity gap among minority women and those who fall within a lower socioeconomic status, ensuring all women have equal, fair, and early access to cancer prevention screening.

REFERENCES

1. Siegel RL, Miller KD, Jemal A. Cancer statistics, 2019. CA Cancer J Clin 2019; 69:7–34.
2. Breast cancer risk assessment and screening in average-risk women. Practice Bulletin No. 179. American College of Obstetricians and Gynecologists. Obstet Gynecol 2017;130:e1–16.
3. Coates RJ, Uhler RJ, Brogan DJ, et al. Patterns and predictors of the breast cancer detection methods in women under 45 years of age (United States). Cancer Causes Control 2001;12:431–4.

4. Nelson HD, Pappas M, Cantor A, et al. Harms of breast cancer screening: system-screening programme. Fam Cancer 2014;13:189–96.

5. Henderson TO, Amsterdam A, Bhatia S, et al. Systemic review: surveillance for breast cancer in women treated with chest radiation for childhood, adolescent, or young adult cancer. Ann Intern Med 2010;152:444–55. W144-W154.

6. Management of women with dense breasts diagnosed by mammography. Committee Opinion No. 625. American College of Obstetricians and Gynecologists. Obstet Gynecol 2015;125:750–1.

7. Dyrstad SW, Yan Y, Fowler AM, et al. Breast cancer risk associated with benign breast diseases: systematic review and meta-analysis. Breast Cancer Res Treat 2015;149:569–75.

8. Hoover RN, Hyer M, Pfeiffer RM, et al. Adverse health outcomes in women exposed in utero to diethylstibestrol. N Engl J Med 2011;365(14):1304–14.

9. Hereditary breast and ovarian cancer syndrome. Practice Bulletin No. 182. American College of Obstetricians and Gynecologists. Obstet Gynecol 2017;130:e110–26.

10. Gibb RK, Martens MG. The impact of liquid-based cytology in decreasing the incidence of cervical cancer. Rev Obstet Gynecol 2011;4(Suppl 1):S2–11.

11. Cervical cancer screening and prevention. Practice Bulletin No. 168. American College of Obstetricians and Gynecologists. Obstet Gynecol 2016;128:e111–30.

12. Saslow D, Solomon D, Lawson HW, et al, ACS-ASCCP-ASCP Cervical Cancer Guideline Committee. American Cancer Society, American Society for Colposcopy and Cervical Pathology and American Society for Clinical Pathology screening guidelines for the prevention and early detection of cervical cancer. CA Cancer J Clin 2012;62:147–72.

13. Huh Wk, Ault KA, Chelmow D, et al. Use of primary high risk human papillomavirus testing for cervical cancer screening: interim clinical guidance. Obstet Gynecol 2015;125:330–7.

14. Curry SJ, Krist AH, Owens DK, et al, US Preventive Services Task Force. Screening for cervical cancer: US preventive services task force recommendation statement. JAMA 2018;320:674–86.

15. Gynecologic care for women and adolescents with human immunodeficiency virus. Practice Bulletin No. 167. American College of Obstetricians and Gynecologists. Obstet Gynecol 2016;128:e89–110.

16. Human papillomavirus vaccination. Committee Opinion No. 704. American College of Obstetricians and Gynecologists. Obstet Gynecol 2017;129:e173–8.

17. Food and Drug Administration. FDA approves expanded use of Gardasil 9 to include individuals 27 through 45 years old [press release]. Silver Spring (MD): FDA; 2018. Available at: https://www.fda.gov/NewsEvents/Newsroom/PressAnnouncements/ucm622715.html.

18. Berian JR, Benson AB, Nelson H. Young age and aggressive treatment in colon cancer. JAMA 2015;314(6):613–4.

19. ACOG District II. Colorectal cancer Task force: focus on female cancers. 2010. Available at: https://www.acog.org/-/media/Districts/District-II/Members Only/PDFs/ColorectalCaChapter.pdf?dmc=1&ts=20190118T1552021627. Accessed January 18, 2019.

20. American Cancer Society. Colorectal cancer screening for average-risk adults: 2018 guideline update from the American Cancer Society. Available at: https://onlinelibrary.wiley.com/doi/abs/10.3322/caac.21457. Accessed January 18 2019.

21. U.S. Preventive Services Task Force. Final recommendation Statement: colorectal cancer: screening. 2017. Available at: https://www.uspreventiveservicestaskforce.

org/Page/Document/RecommendationStatementFinal/colorectal-cancer-screening2. Accessed January 18, 2019.

22. Rex DK, Boland CR, Dominitz JA, et al. Robertson colorectal cancer screening: recommendations for physicians and patients from the U.S. Multi-Society Task Force on Colorectal Cancer. Am J Gastroenterol 2017;112(7):1016.

23. U.S. Preventive Services Task Force. Final recommendation Statement: lung cancer: screening. 2016. Available at: https://www.uspreventiveservicestaskforce. org/Page/Document/RecommendationStatementFinal/lung-cancer-screening. Accessed January 18, 2019.

24. National Lung Screening Trial Research Team, Aberle DR, Adams AM, Berg CD, et al. Reduced lung-cancer mortality with low-dose computed tomographic screening. N Engl J Med 2011;365(5):395.

25. Mazzone PJ, Silvestri GA, Patel S, et al. Screening for lung cancer: CHEST guideline and expert panel report. Chest 2018;153(4):954–85.

26. U.S. Preventive Services Task Force. Draft update summary: lung cancer: screening. 2018. Available at: https://www.uspreventiveservicestaskforce.org/Page/Document/UpdateSummaryDraft/lung-cancer-screening1. Accessed January 18, 2019.

27. U.S. Preventive Services Task Force. Final recommendation Statement: tobacco smoking cessation in adults, including pregnant women: behavioral and pharmacotherapy interventions. 2017. Available at: https://www.uspreventiveservicestaskforce.org/Page/Document/RecommendationStatementFinal/tobacco-use-in-adults-and-pregnant-women-counseling-and-interventions1. Accessed January 18, 2019.

28. Howlader N, Noone AM, Krapcho M, et al. SEER Cancer Statistics Review, 1975-2016. Bethesda (MD): National Cancer Institute. Available at: https://seer.cancer. gov/csr/1975_2016/, based on November 2018 SEER data submission, posted to the SEER web site, April 2019.

29. Jacobs IJ, Menon U, Ryan A, et al. Ovarian cancer screening and mortality in the UK Collaborative Trial of Ovarian Cancer Screening (UKCTOCS): a randomized controlled trial. Lancet 2016;387:945–56.

30. The role of the obstetrician-gynecologist in the early detection of epithelial ovarian cancer in women at average risk. Committee Opinion No. 716. American College of Obstetricians and Gynecologists. Obstet Gynecol 2017;130:e146–9.

31. NCCN Clinical Practice Guidelines in Oncology (NCCN Guidelines). Genetic/familial high-risk assessment: breast and ovarian. Version3.2019. Available at: https://www. nccn.org/professionals/physician_gls/pdf/genetics_screening.pdf. Accessed January 17, 2019.

32. American Cancer Society. Talcum powder and cancer. 2018. Available at: https:// www.cancer.org/cancer/cancer-causes/talcum-powder-and-cancer.html. Accessed March 8, 2019.

Section 2: Maturity

Menopause
Hormones, Lifestyle, and Optimizing Aging

Mary Jane Minkin, MD, NCMP

KEYWORDS

- Menopause • Hormone therapy • GSM • Genitourinary syndrome of menopause
- Vasomotor symptoms

KEY POINTS

- The average age of menopause is 51.5 years in the United States. Twenty percent of women have essentially no symptoms, and 20% of women have severe symptoms. One percent of women are menopausal by age 40, and 5% by age 45.
- Classic symptoms include hot flashes (usually early on) and vulvovaginal atrophic symptoms, classically later on. Many women and providers do not recognize atypical symptoms, such as diffuse achiness.
- Hormonal therapy is the most effective intervention for symptomatic relief. Considerable controversy over estrogen usage has occurred over the past 17 years, with major rethinking on the topic over the past 2 years.
- Nonhormonal therapies and topical hormonal therapies are also available for women with symptoms who cannot take or prefer to avoid systemic hormone therapies.

Menopause marks a major transition in women's lives. The definition of menopause, 12 months of amenorrhea (without any other explanations), signifies the end of a woman's reproductive capacity. For many women, this change is liberating, freeing them from anxieties about childbearing, and from pain or discomfort related to their reproductive organs. Some women may view menopause negatively, associating it with aging, which in most Western cultures has significant negative connotations.

However it is viewed, the menopausal transition is accompanied by a multitude of symptoms and health considerations that may affect all women. The introduction of the first hormonal therapy for menopausal symptoms in 1942 forever changed the landscape of menopause. First thought to be a panacea, estrogen by the 1960s was being touted as a vital substance for all women (Dr Robert Wilson's *Feminine Forever*);[1] however, prescriptions for estrogen have gone through substantial shifts over the past 75 years.[1]

Disclosures: Consultant to Pfizer, AMAG pharmaceuticals, Duchesnay.
Department of Obstetrics, Gynecology and Reproductive Sciences, Yale University School of Medicine, 40 Temple Street, Suite 7A, New Haven, CT 06510, USA
E-mail address: Maryjane.minkin@yale.edu

Obstet Gynecol Clin N Am 46 (2019) 501–514
https://doi.org/10.1016/j.ogc.2019.04.008
0889-8545/19/© 2019 Elsevier Inc. All rights reserved.

Unfortunately, one of the major milestones in hormone therapy history that occurred in 2002 has radically altered clinicians' and patients' comfort with the use of such therapy. The publication of the first set of results from the Women's Health Initiative (WHI) dramatically changed the hormonal landscape. Since that time, the use of menopausal hormonal therapy has declined 80%.[2] Concomitantly, a recent survey of obstetrics and gynecology residents noted that only 21% of their programs had a formal menopause learning curriculum, with 16% reporting a defined menopause clinic as part of their residency.[3] As a result, in the absence of further education, continuity of care for women transitioning through menopause will be jeopardized.

This article aims to fulfill 2 interrelated purposes. First, the author proposes to fill in considerable background for clinicians who have not received adequate menopausal training, and to update everyone on the current state of menopause management for both symptomatic and asymptomatic women. Second, because multiple recent studies indicate that a careful reexamination and reinterpretation of the WHI analyses is required, the author provides a present day perspective on these findings.

Finally, as a stylistic note, in an attempt to best reach a diverse readership, the author has written the core content for ready accessibility, readability, and direct implementation by clinicians. In the same spirit, the author has provided a streamlined minimalist set of references as critical pointers; these, in turn, provide greater specific range so that more specialized readers can find further depth in topics of interest.

DEFINITIONS

Menopause is defined in the first paragraph of this article. The average age of menopause in the United States is between 51 and 52. One percent of women will be fully menopausal by age 40; 5% will be menopausal by age 45. Most women will be fully finished with menses by age 60. Given the prolongation in women's life expectancies, women will be spending 30% to 40% of their lives postmenopausal (contrast this to the year 1900: the average age at menopause was 48, which was also the average female life expectancy).[4]

The concept and timing of perimenopause is much more difficult to define. Most experts will define it as up to 3 years before the final menstrual period and including the first 2 years after the final period; indeed, it is really a retrospective diagnosis. Women are usually alerted by significant menstrual irregularity, and potentially with all the other symptoms of menopause. Many patients mistakenly believe that once they achieve their last period their symptoms will all resolve; much of our responsibility as clinicians is to educate the patients to have realistic expectations. There is no "test" for perimenopause. Most commonly, practitioners will draw a follicle-stimulating hormone (FSH) and estradiol level; however, although abnormal levels (high FSH and low estradiol) may suggest that the patient is in the perimenopausal transition, they do not certify that the last period has arrived, nor that symptoms are likely to abate soon.

SYMPTOMATOLOGY

One of the greatest challenges to clinicians is that although there are classic "menopause symptoms," there is no classic patient. As we go through the menopause transition, we are also getting older, and there is a significant overlap between symptoms occurring with aging and symptoms related to a loss of estrogen. Several major studies have and are examining the components. Among the classic studies are the Melbourne Midlife Women's Study,[5] and the Penn Ovarian Aging study.[6] By enrolling volunteers in their early 40s who were still menstruating, investigators annually studied participants, querying them on various symptoms (such as hot flashes and arthritic symptoms) and also asking about menstrual changes, and measuring various hormonal levels.

From these studies, it has become generally accepted that vasomotor symptoms (hot flashes and night sweats), sleep disruption, and vaginal dryness are mostly related to a loss of estrogen. Most other symptoms have at least a significant component related to aging.

The other components that need to be addressed are the psychosocial issues facing women in their 40s and 50s. Many are dealing with children leaving home, or returning; challenges in the work force to women getting older; partner issues, related to work and to the relationship itself; and the ever-increasing burden of taking care of older relatives, including parents and in-laws. For example, a woman complaining of depression may indeed be a woman with a history of depression, which does increase her likelihood of a menopausal recurrence. However, many life stressors may be presenting concomitantly, and a confusing picture may emerge.[1]

SPECIFIC SYMPTOMS
Vasomotor Symptoms

Hot flashes and night sweats are the most commonly recognized menopausal symptoms in the United States. They can start many years before the final menstrual period. Twenty percent of women will experience severe hot flashes, defined as being accompanied by sweating and stopping the woman's activity. Sixty percent of women will have moderate hot flashes, producing sweating but allowing the continuation of their activity. Twenty percent of women have no or minimal hot flashes; their levels of estrogen are comparable to the women with more severe varieties. In studies examining interventions for hot flashes, qualifying women experience 7 or more moderate to severe flashes daily, or 50 a week.[4]

Hot flashes do tend to improve over the course of time; however, 10% to 15% of women are still experiencing moderate to severe symptoms 10 or more years postmenopausal. The mechanism of the hot flash is not totally understood. It is believed that the thermoregulatory zone in the hypothalamus is narrowed with the loss of estrogen, and that estrogen administration helps to widen it. Current research is also looking at receptors of neurokinin-B as being involved with temperature regulation, with chemical inhibition blocking hot flashes.

Hot flashes are seen with different intensity in different populations. In the Study of Women's Health across the Nation (SWAN Study), performed in the United States, women of different ethnicities had significantly different burdens of vasomotor symptoms, with African American women associated with the highest level, followed by white Hispanic and non Hispanic women, followed by women of Asian backgrounds.[7]

Loss of sleep often accompanies night sweats; however, studies are equivocal as to whether a hot flash will awaken a sleeping woman or whether she will wake up spontaneously and then experience the hot flash.

Urogenital Symptoms

Genital dryness tends to occur later on in the menopausal transition. As hot flashes tend to appear earlier and get better over the course of time, vaginal dryness tends to get worse. Originally referred to as vulvovaginal atrophy, these changes are now termed "the genitourinary syndrome of menopause." Many women found the term atrophic as pejorative; and with the term GUSM or GSM, the bladder is appropriately included in symptoms. In Drs Meadow Maze Good and Ellen R. Solomon's article, "Pelvic Floor Disorders," elsewhere in this issue, points out that many women with pelvic floor disorders think that incontinence and prolapse are a normal consequence of aging.

Vaginal symptoms can include dryness, dyspareunia, and burning. Urinary symptoms can include recurrent urinary tract infections, incontinence, and prolapse.

Urogenital symptoms can be addressed by topical over-the-counter interventions, and topical hormonal therapy. They also may be dealt with by systemic hormonal or selective estrogen receptor modulator (SERM) therapy.[8]

Decrease in Libido

Many women do experience a decrease in libido at the time of menopause. This is one symptom that is truly multifactorial. Dyspareunia contributes to loss of interest in sex for many women; this can be readily dealt with, as described previously. However, there are multiple other factors that potentially contribute. In a practitioner-patient dynamic, an ubiquity question, such as "Many women at the time of menopause have a decrease in libido; is that a problem for you?" can make issues much easier for the woman to bring up. Studies have shown that women feel more comfortable when the provider initiates a discussion of sexual issues with them, and studies have also shown that these are seldom brought up.

There is a very limited choice in potential pharmacologic agents to help increase libido; although testosterone has been shown to be efficacious in such settings, there is no formulation approved by the Food and Drug Administration (FDA) for women in the United States. Flibanserin has been approved for premenopausal women, although there are data showing some efficacy in postmenopausal women. A newer product, bremelanotide, a peptide melanocortin receptor agonist, is currently being reviewed by the FDA for female sexual dysfunction.[9]

Mood Swings, Cognitive Symptoms, and Depression

There is considerable controversy on the prevalence of central nervous system–related symptoms. Many women will complain of some or all of these symptoms, and there is controversy on the role of hormonal therapy in treating them all. As noted previously, exogenous stressors and aging issues also can contribute to these problems.

If a woman has a history of previous depression, the menopause transition can certainly lead to a recurrence of symptoms. It also has been shown that for women suffering from cognitive issues and mood swings, the perimenopausal time frame seems worst for these changes. As women progress further beyond the transition time, these changes seem to resolve. Sleep deprivation can exacerbate any of these symptoms, and therapies to ameliorate sleeping patterns can be very helpful.

Achiness

Women also complain of generalized musculoskeletal achiness. In some populations, this is the major menopausal complaint (eg, in the Philippines). Many women experiencing achiness will present for an annual visit after a full evaluation by a rheumatologist, and with all blood tests indicating no evidence of collagen vascular diseases. A significant percentage of these women will respond to hormonal therapy. This achiness is unrelated to bone loss.

Weight Gain

Most women complain of weight gain in the menopausal transition. Animal studies confirm that the loss of estrogen can contribute to weight gain and fat redistribution, with the tendency to gain weight in the abdominal area. The etiology is complex, in that many women are less active and lose muscle mass, further complicating an explanation of the weight gain. Women may gain approximately 5 to 8 pounds in the menopausal transition. However, once a woman is fully menopausal, further weight gain attributable to menopause should cease.

Skin and Hair Changes

Most women note significant skin dryness as they enter menopause. Many women also complain about hair loss. Although these are not considered classic menopausal symptoms, many women will opt for systemic therapy to combat these dermatologic issues. Any woman complaining of these symptoms should be evaluated with a thyroid-stimulating hormone evaluation to rule out hypothyroidism.

Asymptomatic Health Considerations Associated with Menopause

Even if a menopausal patient comes in for her annual visit with no complaints, there are still health considerations that require attention. Both cardiovascular disease and bone loss are associated with the loss of estrogen, beyond the risks attendant with regular aging. If a woman is not seeing a primary care physician regularly, she should be assessed for cardiovascular risk factors (family history, weight, diabetes, smoking, and exercise habits, and from her obstetric history, a history of preeclampsia). Find out when her last lipid profile was done, and update if needed. Loss of estrogen has been associated with an elevation of low-density lipoprotein and triglycerides. If investigation indicates problems that would not routinely be handled by a gynecologist, the patient should be referred to a specialist.

Although current guidelines do not recommend a routine bone density when a patient becomes menopausal, routine care should include an assessment for risk factors for bone loss. The risk factors are well-covered by Dr Carolyn J. Crandall's article, "Strong Bones, Strong Body," in on bone health elsewhere in this issue. All women should have a bone density at age 65. Major risk factors include history of previous fractures, family history of osteoporosis, low weight (under 127 pounds), smoking, history of corticosteroid use, and previous history of long periods of amenorrhea. If the patient has 1 or more of these risk factors, it may be appropriate to establish a baseline bone density before age 65.

All women should be apprised of the need for good bone health habits. All women should be counseled on vitamin D and calcium intake (ideally with most calcium being consumed from food sources as opposed to supplements). Most women should be taking at least 800 IU daily of vitamin D. Most women (barring contraindications such as history of certain types of kidney stones) should aim to take in approximately 1200 mg of calcium daily. Weight-bearing exercises should be emphasized. Counseling on smoking cessation should be offered.[8]

MANAGEMENT OF MENOPAUSAL SYMPTOMATOLOGY

This section focuses on management of the major menopausal issues definitively related to the loss of estrogen: namely, vasomotor symptoms and GSM. First, the focus is on nonmedical (nonprescription) interventions, and then guidelines for hormonal interventions, as well as nonhormonal medications, are discussed.

Many basic measures may not be known by patients. Simple advice on layered dressing, for example, wearing a shell underneath a sweater, gives women a bit more control over their environment. Keeping a bedroom cool at night, especially during the first 4 hours of sleep, promotes less disrupted sleep. Cooling pillows may help.

Keeping a dry set of night clothes next to a bed will help her if she gets up soaking in sweat.[1]

Avoiding known hot flash triggers usually helps. Classic triggers include hot beverages, spicy foods, and red wine. More broadly, many women will turn to alcohol to help them sleep; this is usually counterproductive, in that it promotes a more disruptive sleep pattern, and exacerbates hot flashes.

Many women believe that certain herbal products and vitamins may help prevent hot flashes. Very few products have been evaluated by prospective randomized double-blinded studies; and herbal products in the United States vary significantly in components so that large randomized trials across many preparations are very difficult to perform. All trials for hot flash relief show a very large placebo effect of at least 35%. Any study of a product for VMS requires a placebo arm.

The role of soy is controversial. Soy contains weak plant estrogens called isoflavones. There are limited studies that show that soy in the diet may help hot flashes. The effect is modest. However, the central question in the literature is whether soy isoflavones also stimulate breast tissue. Again, the topic is quite controversial. Some in the oncology community think that soy is thus somewhat risky; however, many believe that soy may have SERM-like properties, protecting the breast from stimulation by a more potent estrogen. In general, soy in moderation is reasonable. Nonetheless, if a woman is being monitored for breast disease risk by an oncologist, the woman should inform her treating physician of the degree (if any) of soy use.[8]

Prescription Nonhormonal Therapy

There are 2 current mainstays for nonhormonal therapy for vasomotor symptoms. Selective serotonin reuptake inhibitors (SSRIs) and selective norepinephrine reuptake inhibitors (SNRIs) have both been shown to help relieve hot flashes. Small doses, even lower than antidepressant dosing, can be helpful. There is currently 1 SSRI product (paroxetine, 7.5 mg) that is FDA approved for vasomotor symptoms. The use of all others is off-label. Given the potential side-effect profile of SSRIs and SNRIs, namely weight gain and loss of libido, the use of these medications must be monitored closely to maximize benefit while minimizing adverse reactions.

The other nonhormonal (and off-label) option is gabapentin. Again, used in much lower doses than for neurologic indications, it can be effective for hot flash relief. Given the potential side effect of sedation, it is usually prescribed before bed, starting at a small dose; a level of 300 mg is usually tolerated. The other side effect is bloating, which again must be monitored in menopausal women.[8]

Hormonal Therapy

The most comprehensive and up-to-date summary of hormone therapy is the 2017 hormone therapy position statement of the North American Menopause Society (NAMS).[10] We summarize their recommendations based on an extensive review of evidence. Readers are referred to the article in *Menopause*[10] and to references indicated. Most of the international societies have endorsed the NAMS guidelines. "The American College of Obstetricians and Gynecologists supports the value of this clinical document as an educational tool, June 2017."[10]

The author states, "Hormone therapy [HT] remains the most effective treatment for vasomotor symptoms and genitourinary syndrome of menopause and has been shown to prevent bone loss and fracture. The risks of HT differ depending on type, dose, duration of use, route of administration, timing of initiation, and whether progestogen is used. Treatment should be individualized to identify the most appropriate HT type, dose, formulation, route of administration, and duration of use, using the best available evidence to maximize the benefits and minimize the risks, with periodic reevaluation of the benefits and risks of continuing or discontinuing HT."[10]

These recommendations are in stark contrast to the original interpretations of the WHI findings, which had 2 arms. In the estrogen/progestin arm, only 1 preparation was investigated, namely oral conjugated estrogens plus medroxyprogesterone acetate, 0.625 mg/2.5 mg. In the estrogen-only arm, for hysterectomized women, only conjugated estrogen 0.625 mg was investigated. Yet when the FDA considered the findings of the WHI, boxed warnings were issued for all women, and stated to pertain to all estrogens and progestogens, and to all doses and routes of administration. The study group for the WHI was woman aged 50 to 79, which in general is not the typical group for whom we initiate hormone therapy. Indeed, the purpose of the WHI was to investigate the question, "Does hormone therapy help prevent coronary artery disease?" The study was never intended to be a study of side effects of hormonal therapy for symptomatic women.[10,11] To reinforce this point, WHI investigator and WHI steering committee member Drs JoAnn Manson and Andrew Kaunitz have noted, "its results are now being used inappropriately in making decisions about treatment for women in their 40s and 50s who have distressing vasomotor symptoms."[12]

BASIC CLINICAL GUIDELINES
Estrogens (Systemic Forms)

Two basic oral estrogens are available in the United States: conjugated estrogens and 17 beta estradiol. The conjugated equine estrogen (CEE) used in the WHI is actually a mixture of more than 10 forms of estrogen. The biological activity of 1 mg of estradiol is approximately equivalent to that of 0.625 mg of CEE. There are no direct comparative studies of estradiol to CEE, including any safety comparisons.

All transdermal forms of estrogen are estradiol; these include patches, gels, and sprays. One vaginal ring (Femring) is available that delivers estradiol in a high enough dosage to achieve systemic levels.

The major contraindications to systemic estrogen in any form are unexplained vaginal bleeding, severe active liver disease, coronary heart disease, previous breast cancer, dementia, personal history of thromboembolic disease, and hypertriglyceridemia. Relative concerns would include reactivation of endometriosis or growth of fibroids. Gall bladder disease is a known side effect of oral estrogen therapy; the risk seems lower with transdermal estrogens. Fluid retention and breast discomfort are the most common annoying side effects.

Women who have had a hysterectomy do not need to take progestogens with their systemic estrogens. The WHI, among many other studies, has shown that after 7.1 years of estrogen-alone therapy there was a nonsignificant decrease in the diagnosis of breast cancer. There are some observational studies that have suggested that in women who take estrogen therapy for more than 10 years, there may be a slight increased risk of being diagnosed with breast cancer; others have not shown such a risk.

The major health risk shown in the WHI with oral estrogens was an increased risk of thromboembolic events. European studies have suggested in observational trials that transdermal estrogens do not increase the risk of thromboembolic events (consistent with bypassing the first pass effect through the liver, and no significant effect on clotting factors.) There are no prospective randomized trials. Vaginal estrogens do not increase the risk of thromboembolic phenomena.[13]

Progestogens

Women who have their uterus in place need to take a progestogen with their systemic estrogen to reduce the risk for development of endometrial hyperplasia or cancer. Traditional synthetic progestins, such as MPA (medroxyprogesterone acetate), norethindrone, and drospirenone are all available in oral forms. Some are available as part of transdermal patch systems. An intrauterine device containing levonorgestrel also can serve to deliver the protective progestin. Micronized natural progesterone (FDA approved) also is available, in both oral and vaginal forms.

Another option available to women is the combination of estrogen with an SERM. The SERM bazedoxifene combined with estrogen, in appropriate dosing, can effectively provide endometrial protection. Use of bazedoxifene may be helpful for women who cannot tolerate progestin side effects. In the United States, bazedoxifene is currently available only with conjugated estrogens in 1 pill and 1 dosage level.

Therapies including progestogens include both daily administration of the progestin, and cyclic regimens. Daily regimens are easy to remember. However, daily regimens are associated with a significant rate of breakthrough bleeding (BTB), and the more proximate to the last menstrual bleed, the greater likelihood of BTB. Many women eventually will achieve reasonably rapid amenorrhea with this regimen. Cyclic progestin usually at least initially produces withdrawal bleeding; but the rate of unscheduled bleeding is lower.

Progestogen therapies can be associated with annoying side effects for your patients. Besides the bleeding issues, progestins can induce mood swings and breast tenderness, with MPA being the most likely to induce side effects and natural progesterone the least.

From a health perspective, the major concerning side effect associated with long-term progestin therapy is a slight increased risk of being diagnosed with breast cancer. In the WHI, after 5.5 years of continuous combined conjugated estrogen and MPA, the hazard ratio of being diagnosed with breast cancer was 1.24 (confidence interval 1.01–1.53). The attributable risk was 8 per 10,000 women per year. This number and the attendant publicity was the primary cause of the rapid decline in use of hormone therapy in the United States. (This attributable risk is actually less than that associated with ingestion of 2 glasses of wine daily.) Of note is that in the 18-year follow-up of the WHI, no increase in mortality was noted from breast cancer.[14]

Indeed, published data on the role of hormone therapy and the risk of ovarian cancer are conflicting.[8] It is not clear if hormone therapy increases risk. The studies that have shown a slight increased risk have been large observational trials, and not randomized controlled trials. The WHI E plus P study did not show any statistically significant increased risk.

In case control studies from Europe, micronized natural progesterone (combined with estrogen) has been shown to have a minimal, if any, risk of breast cancer with long-term therapy. There are no prospective randomized data.[15]

Compounded Hormonal Therapy

After the publication of the WHI, a large industry in compounded "bioidentical hormones" arose. The term bioidentical refers to hormonal therapy that is similar to endogenous hormones 17 beta estradiol and progesterone. Most patients assume that these hormones need to be compounded, and are not available commercially. FDA-approved bioidentical estradiol and progesterone are readily available. Also available only through compounding pharmacies is estriol, which is not approved by the FDA for any use in the United States. There is a common misconception that estriol is safer for use than estradiol; there are no safety data available. Estriol is a very weak estrogen compared with estradiol.

NAMS strongly recommends that "prescribers should only consider compounded HT [hormone therapy] if women cannot tolerate a government-approved therapy for reasons such as allergies to ingredients or for a dose or formulation not currently available in government-approved therapies."[10] One reason patients believe compounded therapy to be safer than commercially available products is that the compounded products are not mandated to be provided with a patient insert from the FDA; as a consequence, many patients assume these products have no side effects associated with their use.[10] Some women have been led to believe that because there are no large studies on compounded hormones, they are safer than the commercially available hormones. That is untrue.

Many of the providers who prescribe compounded therapy rely on salivary hormonal testing, which has been shown to be "unreliable because of differences in hormone pharmacokinetics and absorption, diurnal variation, and interindividual and intraindividual variability."[10]

Androgen Therapy

Unfortunately, there is no FDA-approved form of testosterone available in dosages appropriate for women. Therefore, if one is prescribing testosterone, one needs to rely on compounding pharmacies.

NAMS recommendations for clinical care from 2014 do address androgen therapy. Women with surgical menopause and primary ovarian insufficiency are known to have significantly lower levels of androgens. They do endorse the use of testosterone in "carefully selected postmenopausal women with female sexual interest/arousal disorder, and no other identified etiology for their sexual problem."[4] However, they do note that long-term risks of androgen therapy in women, particularly regarding cardiovascular disease and breast cancer, are not known. Certain side effects are well known, including facial hair, acne, voice changes, and clitoromegaly, as well as lipid and liver function test abnormalities. They do recommend periodically checking blood testosterone levels even though low levels of testosterone achieved in women are not totally accurate.[4]

Vaginal Therapy

Many women will have tried over-the-counter remedies for GSM before consulting their gynecologist; conversely, many will not be aware of them. As mentioned previously, women often need to be reminded about the availability of both lubricants to be used primarily at the time of intercourse, and longer-acting moisturizers to be used on an ongoing basis. The longer-acting products are usually composed of either a polycarbophil or hyaluronic acid, to draw fluid into the vaginal wall. However, if a patient has had insufficient relief from the over-the-counter regimens, and particularly if she is suffering from urinary issues, she may well need prescription interventions.

Vaginal estrogens are available as creams, vaginal tablets or suppositories, and rings. The creams may be used both internally for vaginal symptoms and externally for vulvar issues. The tablets and rings work well for internal symptoms. When used in appropriate dosages, there is minimal systemic absorption. The vaginal ring is kept in continuously, and needs to be changed every 3 months. The other products are usually initiated with daily therapy for 2 weeks, after which usage is switched to a twice weekly regimen.

There are no data that suggest that women using vaginal estrogen therapy need to use any progestins for endometrial protection. If a woman exhibits vaginal bleeding, she should be evaluated, as any postmenopausal woman should.

More recent introductions to our armamentarium include topical dehydroepiandrosterone (DHEA), called prasterone. It is administered nightly as a vaginal suppository. Mechanism of action is through intracrine metabolism of DHEA in the vaginal cells to both estrogens and androgens, with further local breakdown leading to minimal systemic absorption.[16]

None of the vaginal therapies are associated with any significant systemic absorption; accordingly, both the American College of Obstetricians and Gynecologists (ACOG) and NAMS approved use of these products in breast cancer survivors. However, there are no long-term trials available of use of any products and risk of recurrent disease.[17,18]

Systemic estrogen therapy will alleviate symptoms of GSM for most women; however, approximately 20% may need a vaginal "booster," particularly with low systemic doses.

There is one oral nonestrogen therapy available for GSM. It is the oral SERM ospemifene. Ospemifene blocks estrogen activity in the breast, as do all SERMs; however, at the vagina, ospemifene binds to the estrogen receptors and stimulates moisture. Taken once daily with food, it helps alleviate dyspareunia.

Should Hormonal Therapy Be Prescribed for Prevention of Chronic Diseases?

The WHI was intended as a study to evaluate the use of hormone replacement therapy for prevention of coronary heart disease. For the age range studied, namely women 50 to 79, the WHI demonstrated that it did not prevent coronary heart disease (CHD). The official recommendation of the US Preventive Services Task Force, issued in 2017, for women with and without a uterus, was that they "recommended against the use of HT [hormone therapy] for the primary prevention of chronic conditions in postmenopausal women."[19]

However, the final recommendation statement notes that it does not apply "to women who are considering hormone therapy for the management of menopausal symptoms such as hot flashes and vaginal dryness."[19] From a preventive medicine perspective, "it does not apply to women who have had premature menopause (primary ovarian insufficiency) or surgical menopause." A commentary from the European Menopause and Andropause Society emphasizes the latter group, noting "that premature menopause is associated with an increased risk of osteoporotic fractures, cardiovascular disease, etc."[20]

The NAMS (hormone therapy) position statement notes that women with premature menopause "who require prevention of bone loss are best served with HT [hormone therapy]"[10] rather than "other bone-specific treatments until the average age of menopause."[10] The position statement also notes, "For women with POI [premature ovarian insufficiency] or premature surgical menopause without contraindications, HT is recommended until at least the median age of menopause (52 y) because observational studies suggest that benefits outweigh the risks for effects on bone, heart, cognitions, GSM, sexual function and mood."[10]

Recently there has been an emergent generation of women with premature menopause, namely BRCA-positive women who are undergoing prophylactic bilateral salpingo-oophorectomies in their 30s. In the women who have no cancer diagnosis, also known as "previvors," good observational trials do show that there is no increased risk of cancer diagnoses in these young women given hormonal replacement therapy.[21]

What Is the Current Interpretation of Cardiac Risk Associated with Hormone Therapy?

As noted previously, the WHI was undertaken to ask the question "Does estrogen therapy decrease the risk of cardiovascular disease in women?" Studies started appearing in the 1980s indicating that women who took estrogen therapy for menopausal symptomatology experienced a dramatic reduction in cardiac disease. Typical women initiating therapy were in their 40s and early 50s. Although the WHI did include some early menopausal women as participants, the average age of women in the WHI was 63, typically many years after menopause. Twenty percent of the women in the WHI were aged 70 to 79 on enrollment.[11]

It is this "gap time" that is offered as the most likely explanation of the differences in the cardiac effects noted between the observational studies and the WHI. Much earlier primate studies had suggested such an outcome.[22] One study performed subsequently to investigate this hypothesis in humans was the Early versus Late Intervention Trial with Estradiol (ELITE) trial.[23] The ELITE trial used as a surrogate marker for cardiovascular disease the carotid artery intima-media thickness (CIMT). In women started on hormone therapy less than 6 years after menopause, decreased thickening of the CIMT was shown. However, in women started on hormone therapy 10 years or more after menopause, no such benefit was noted. Other trials have reported similar results.

Currently, most cardiologists believe that hormonal therapy started proximate to menopause is quite safe; however, if a woman is many years postmenopausal, it would be prudent to consult a menopause specialist on potential risks. The HERS trial (Heart and Estrogen/progestin Replacement Study) examined the prophylactic use of hormonal therapy in women with established coronary artery disease. The investigators showed that there were no significant differences between treated and control groups in primary outcome (myocardial infarction or CHD death) or in any secondary cardiovascular outcomes. Indeed, the analyses suggested that in the long-term, the treated women were slightly more likely to have *fewer* adverse cardiac events than were the women in the control group over the study duration. Thus, we readily infer that women already on therapy with cardiovascular disease could continue usage of hormonal therapy.[24]

General Hormonal Therapy Guidelines for Cancer Survivors

With the welcome improvement in all forms of cancer therapies, there are burgeoning numbers of cancer survivors. We have alluded to some of the issues earlier in this article. Both ACOG and NAMS have opined that vaginal hormonal therapy is safe for breast cancer survivors, because of the very minimal systemic absorption from these products. These recommendations are usually applied to nearly all cancer survivors, including gynecologic cancer survivors. Certain cancer survivors, such as rectal cancer survivors, are particularly vulnerable to pelvic scarring from pelvic radiation. Most of these women will benefit from GSM therapy.

Concerning the questions on systemic hormone therapy, many cancers have no estrogen receptors. Women who have had hematological or lung cancers are often excellent candidates for systemic therapy. One consideration that may be helpful is to use a transdermal estrogen preparation, for the observational finding that these formulations are less likely to increase any thromboembolic risk.

Most medical oncologists will not allow their patients with breast cancer to use systemic estrogen therapy. If there is a question on an individual basis, these patients would be best referred to a menopause specialist. However, most patients with gynecologic cancer are reasonable candidates for hormonal therapy. Even women with stage 1 and 2 endometrial cancers are usually considered reasonable candidates for systemic therapy, although there is not abundant prospective randomized data.[25]

Duration of Therapy

There is no exact formula applicable to all women on how long to continue hormonal therapy. The major cancer risk is the very slight increased risk of breast cancer seen with hormonal therapy for many years. The major chronic disease–related benefit will be ongoing bone protection, which persists as long as your patient continues her hormonal therapy. Cardiovascular protection is currently a hotly debated topic. As noted previously, there should be no arbitrary cutoff points, and current NAMS guidelines promote individualization of care, using the "appropriate dose for the appropriate duration."[10]

PERSPECTIVE AND FUTURE DIRECTIONS

Many women will go through the menopause transition with minimal complaints. Some will suffer significantly, and many women will experience issues that neither they nor their care providers will associate with menopause. Even for those who escape significant symptomatology, much basic physiology is affected by the loss of estrogen. Hopefully the guidance presented in this article will help educate providers and their patients.

The American Geriatrics Society has recently published the Beers Criteria for potentially inappropriate medication use in older adults, in which they state that "systemic estrogen is a high-risk medication because of its carcinogenic potential and lack of cardiovascular protective effects."[26] Sadly, many insurers will then decline to pay for the cost of hormone therapy for their patients older than 65 based on this statement,[26] which then places an undue burden on many women in their later years. However, ACOG has directly addressed this issue in its Committee Opinion 565, issued in 2013 and reaffirmed in 2018. Specifically, ACOG "recommends against routine discontinuation of systemic estrogen at age 65 years," and instead recommends that "as with younger women, use of HT [hormone therapy] and ET [estrogen therapy] should be individualized based on each woman's risk benefit ratio and clinical presentation."[27] We strongly recommend that the ACOG guidelines be very actively disseminated to insurers, through multiple media and with political pressure, if necessary, to ensure as best as possible, that women have ready access to hormone therapy and estrogen therapy if and when these therapies are required.

In the spirit of optimizing aging, a critically important recommendation for women is not strictly medical: it is the development of a long-term relationship with a fixed provider or group. With the proliferation of health-related propaganda on the Internet, quality-of-life issues need to be discussed with a longstanding and trusted provider.

We can never cease to reinforce the importance of a healthy lifestyle, with proper exercise and nutrition, independent of any pharmacologic advancements. To augment this point somewhat, many recent studies also have established the utility of some strength training as part of one's workout or exercise regimen, for improvement in both long-term cognitive capability and adverse event protection.

As we indicated earlier, the present extent of menopausal education to providers in training is quite inadequate. Accordingly, the development of educational tools and modules is acutely needed, as is enhanced training. Moreover, a delineation of the symptomatology and efficacy of treatment modalities among racial, ethnic, and sexual orientation subgroups is sorely needed, and quite timely.

As a final and overarching viewpoint, the decision of whether and how to use hormonal therapy is truly a paradigm example of the modern terminology of "shared decision making." Science is evolving, and as our patients are living longer, we can all help them to lead healthier and happier lives.

REFERENCES

1. Minkin MJ, Giblin K. Manual of management counseling for the perimenopausal and menopausal patient: a clinician's guide. New York: Parthenon Publishing Group; 2004. p. 1–47.
2. Santen RJ, Stuenkel CA, Burger HG, et al. Competency in menopause management: whither goest the internist? J Womens Health 2014;23:281–5.
3. Christianson MS, Ducie JA, Altman K, et al. Menopause education: needs assessment of American obstetrics and gynecology residents. Menopause 2013;20:1120–5.
4. Shifren JL, Gass ML, for the NAMS Recommendations for Clinical Care of Midlife Women Working Group. The North American Menopause Society recommendations for clinical care of midlife women. Menopause 2014;21:1038–61.
5. Burger HG, Hale GE, Robertson DM, et al. A review of hormonal changes during the menopausal transition: focus on the findings from the Melbourne Women's Midlife Health Project. Hum Reprod Update 2007;13:559–65.
6. Freeman EW, Sammel MD, Lin H, et al. Duration of menopausal hot flushes and associated risk factors. Obstet Gynecol 2011;117:1095–104.
7. Thurston RC, Joffe H. Vasomotor symptoms and menopause: findings from the Study of Women's Health across the Nation. Obstet Gynecol Clin North Am 2011;38:489–501.
8. Allam SA, Allen RH, Bachmann GA, et al. Menopause practice: a clinician's guide. 5th edition. Mayfield Heights (OH): The North American Menopause Society; 2014.
9. Minkin MJ. Sexuality, sexual dysfunction and menopause. In: Pal L, Sayegh RA, editors. Essentials of menopause management. Basel (Switzerland): Springer International Publishing; 2017. p. 165–71.
10. The NAMS 2017 Hormone Therapy Position Statement Advisory Panel. The 2017 hormone therapy position statement of the North American Menopause Society. Menopause 2017;24:728–53.
11. Langer RD. The evidence base for HRT: what can we believe? Climacteric 2017; 20:91–6.
12. Manson JE, Kaunitz AM. Menopause management—getting clinical care back on track. N Engl J Med 2016;374:803–6.
13. Canonico M. Hormone therapy and hemostasis among postmenopausal women: a review. Menopause 2014;21:753–62.
14. Manson JE, Aragaki AK, Rossouw JE, et al. Menopausal hormone therapy and long-term all-cause and cause-specific mortality: the Women's Health Initiative randomized trials. JAMA 2017;318:927–38.
15. Gompel A, Plu-Bureau G. Progesterone, progestins and the breast in menopause treatment. Climacteric 2018;21:326–32.
16. Labrie F, Archer DF, Koltun W, et al. Efficacy of intravaginal dehydroepiandrosterone (DHEA) on moderate to severe dyspareunia and vaginal dryness, symptoms of vulvovaginal atrophy, and of the genitourinary syndrome of menopause. Menopause 2018;25:1339–53.

17. American College of Obstetricians and Gynecologists' Committee on Gynecologic Practice, Farrell R. ACOG Committee opinion no. 659 summary: the use of vaginal estrogen in women with a history of estrogen-dependent breast cancer. Obstet Gynecol 2016;127:618–9.

18. Faubion SS, Larkin LC, Stuenkel CA, et al. Management of genitourinary syndrome of menopause in women with or at high risk for breast cancer: consensus recommendations from the North American Menopause Society and the International Society for the Study of Women's Sexual Health. Menopause 2018;25:1–13.

19. US Preventative Services Task Force, Grossman DC, Curry SJ, Owens DK, et al. Hormone therapy for the primary prevention of chronic conditions in postmenopausal women. US Preventative Services Task Force recommendation statement. JAMA 2017;318:2224–33.

20. Cano A, Rees M, Simoncini T. Comments on the USPSTF draft recommendation statement on menopausal hormone therapy: primary prevention of chronic conditions. Maturitas 2018;107:A1–2.

21. Domchek S, Kaunitz AM. Use of systemic hormone therapy in BRCA mutation carriers. Menopause 2018;23:1026–7.

22. Clarkson TB, Mehaffey MH. Coronary heart disease of females: lessons learned from nonhuman primates. Am J Primatol 2009;71:785–93.

23. Hodis HN, Mack WJ, Henderson VW, et al. Vascular effects of early versus late postmenopausal treatment with estradiol. N Engl J Med 2016;374:1221–31.

24. Hulley S, Grady D, Bush T, et al. Randomized trial of estrogen plus progestin for secondary prevention of coronary heart disease in postmenopausal women. Heart and Estrogen/progestin Replacement Study (HERS) Research Group. JAMA 1998;280:605–13.

25. Kuhle CL, Kapoor E, Sood R, et al. Menopausal hormonal therapy in cancer survivors: a narrative review of the literature. Maturitas 2016;92:86–96.

26. 2015 BEERS Criteria Update Expert Panel. American Geriatrics Society BEERS Criteria for potentially inappropriate medication use in older adults. J Am Geriatr Soc 2015;63:2227–46.

27. ACOG Committee Opinion. Hormone therapy and heart disease. Obstet Gynecol 2013;121:1407–10.

Matters of the Heart
Cardiovascular Health in Women Throughout Their Lifetimes

Rachel A. Newman, MD, MBA[a], Afshan B. Hameed, MD[b],*

KEYWORDS

- Adolescent cardiovascular guidelines • Postpartum cardiovascular screening
- Women's preventive screening • Menopause • HRT and cardiovascular disease

KEY POINTS

- The American Heart Association defines ideal cardiovascular health as having optimal levels of total cholesterol, blood pressure, and fasting glucose as well as being physically active, being a non-smoker, and eating well.
- Risk factors for cardiovascular disease may start to appear as early as adolescence; however, there is no clear consensus on universal screening for adolescents, despite recommendations from the American Academy of Pediatrics and Women's Preventive Screening Initiative.
- Pregnancy is a unique period of life in which the body must adjust to changing cardiovascular demands. Conditions of pregnancy, such a preeclampsia, may increase risk of poor cardiovascular health later in life.
- Depletion of estrogen and variation in hormone levels after menopause can further increase a woman's cardiovascular risk.

INTRODUCTION

The American Heart Association (AHA) defines "ideal cardiovascular health" as the absence of clinical cardiovascular disease (CVD) along with the following:

i. Optimal levels of total cholesterol, blood pressure, and fasting blood glucose,
ii. Body mass index less than 25, and
iii. Healthy behaviors, such as being a non-smoker, being physically active, and adhering to a DASH (Dietary Approaches to Stop Hypertension)-like diet.[1]

Disclosure Statement: The authors have nothing to disclose.
[a] Department of Obstetrics and Gynecology, University of California, Irvine Medical Center, 333 City Boulevard West, 14th Floor, Suite 1400, Orange, CA 92868, USA; [b] Department of Obstetrics and Gynecology, Division of Maternal-Fetal Medicine, University of California, Irvine Medical Center, 333 City Boulevard West, 14th Floor, Suite 1400, Orange, CA 92868, USA
* Corresponding author.
E-mail address: ahameed@uci.edu

The authors' goal is to review the current recommendations for optimizing cardio-vascular health beginning in adolescent years to adulthood and to expand on the role that pregnancy complications may have as implications for future cardiovascular health.

CARDIAC RISK FACTORS IN CHILDHOOD AND ADOLESCENCE

Traditionally, CVD has been considered an affliction of middle and old age. However, CVD may develop and progress over time as evidenced by signs of atherosclerosis as early as adolescence in otherwise healthy individuals.[2] With the increase in prevalence of CVD risk factors across all ages, it is not surprising to witness earlier onset of CVD, and therefore, adolescence provides an opportunity to intervene and establish screening programs that can identify young women at low versus higher risk of future cardiovascular events.

Currently, there is a lack of standardized guidance for assessment of cardiovascular risk in young women. For example, the US Preventive Services Task Force (USPSTF) does not recommend routine CVD screening for adolescents. However, the Women's Preventive Services Initiative (WPSI) recommends blood pressure and lipid screening beginning at age 13 for those with familial dyslipidemia, risk factors, or high-risk con-ditions.[3] Furthermore, the American Academy of Pediatrics recommends that children and adolescents with a family history of dyslipidemia or premature coronary artery dis-ease (<55 years of age for men, <65 years of age for women), or those who have family members with other risk factors for CVD, such as obesity, hypertension, smoking, or diabetes mellitus, should be screened with a fasting lipid profile between ages 2 and 10 years of age.[4]

Many of the strongest risk factors for CVD in adults, such as high low-density lipoprotein (LDL), low high-density lipoprotein (HDL), obesity, and elevated blood pressure, are also found in relatively young individuals.[4,5] Therefore, preventive mea-sures should be started in adolescence. However, because there is no clear guidance, there is little in the way of standardized risk assessment for CVD in younger years. Research has identified the best approach to triage of children and adolescents at risk; however, there remains a wide gap in clinical practice. Some providers rely on a positive family history to guide screening recommendations,[6] whereas others favor universal screening, a preferred strategy that serves this population in a proactive fashion.[3]

Although there is more guidance for specific risk factors that can lead to CVD, the uptake for the recommendations are limited. For example, the USPSTF and National Cholesterol Education Program (NCEP) recommended screening children with a family history of premature coronary artery disease or high blood concentrations of choles-terol.[6,7] The major limitation of this approach is that family history may be unknown, incomplete, or inaccurate, or the adult family members may not have had cholesterol levels assessed.[8] NCEP found that only 35% to 46% of children and adolescents have had their cholesterol checked as a result of a positive family history of CVD or elevated cholesterol.[9,10] Clearly, many children and adolescents are not being screened. Although there is some evidence that adolescents with elevated cholesterol have persistently higher levels of cholesterol in adulthood than the general population, there is a paucity of data suggesting that a certain childhood cholesterol level predicts CVD in adulthood. Therefore, NCEP and the American Academy of Pediatrics recom-mend both population and individual approaches to reducing cholesterol.[4,7]

The nationwide increase in obesity, diabetes, and elevated blood pressure includes children. Evidence shows effective weight management through diet and exercise can decrease the risk of a child developing CVD or diabetes.[11] The AHA recently updated dietary recommendations for children older than 2 years of age, including guidance to consume more fruits, vegetables, fish, whole grains, and low-fat dairy.[12,13] For children with a strong genetic basis for dyslipidemia, including familial hypercholesterolemia, a higher level of dietary intervention may be needed.[7]

Although guidelines for childhood and adolescence cardiac health have yet to be standardized, given that the rates of well-known precursors to cardiac disease, such as type 2 diabetes mellitus and hypertension, continue to increase in the childhood and adolescent years, this is a demographic whose heart health should no longer be ignored.[14,15]

CARDIAC RISK FACTORS IN PREGNANCY

Pregnancy is considered a natural stress test for the maternal cardiovascular system.[16] Pregnancy is a unique period in a woman's life as the body must adjust to meet the altered cardiovascular and metabolic needs of the mother and developing fetus.[17] Failure of the body to do so may be due to impaired organ function, which manifests as disease processes, such as gestational hypertension or preeclampsia.[17,18] Furthermore, the process of labor and delivery with accompanying anxiety, pain, and exertion can place additional stress on the cardiovascular system. Although the body returns to physiologic baseline after delivery, it may be useful to consider conditions that manifest during pregnancy as predictors of future illness.[18]

For example, a large meta-analysis found that women with a history of preeclampsia have approximately double the risk for subsequent ischemic heart disease, stroke, and venous thromboembolic events over the 5 to 15 years after pregnancy.[19] Another recent cohort study found that more than 50 years after pregnancy, cardiovascular outcomes in women with preexisting chronic hypertension with superimposed preeclampsia had an approximately 6-fold increase in cardiovascular events when compared with women who had chronic hypertension alone.[20,21] Clearly, pregnancy and the postpartum period provide a window of opportunity to identify risk factors for women to improve long-term health.[22]

Pregnancy-related cardiovascular risk factors include preeclampsia, eclampsia, HELLP (hemolysis, elevated liver enzymes, low platelet count syndrome), gestational hypertension, gestational diabetes, impaired glucose tolerance, intrauterine growth restriction (<2000 g at term, <5th percentile), idiopathic preterm birth, placental abruption, excessive weight gain in pregnancy, and postpartum weight retention.[19,22–24] Even though the conditions of pregnancy leading to CVD have been identified, there is no universal screening algorithm to assess the risk of a cardiac complication during pregnancy.

The California Maternal Quality Care Collaborative encourages CVD assessment be done for every patient at some point in time during pregnancy and/or the postpartum period to prevent maternal mortality because CVD is the number 1 cause of indirect maternal death in the United States.[25] The CVD in pregnancy toolkit includes an algorithm that would have identified 93% of the women who died as being high risk of CVD and perhaps would have altered outcomes (**Fig. 1**). Validation studies are currently underway.

It is well studied that women with a history of hypertensive disorders of pregnancy have an increased risk of future cardiovascular events.[26] A general risk calculator, such as the Framingham Risk Score, is inadequate because the initial 10-year score incorporates a protective benefit for those who are young women.[22] As a result, the score

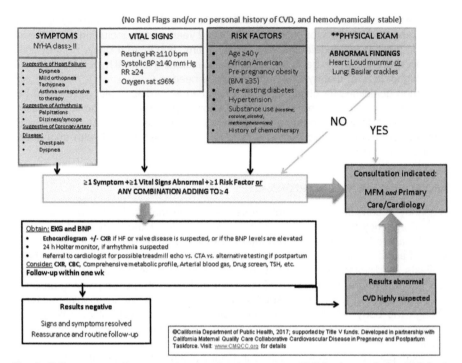

Fig. 1. CVD assessment in pregnant and postpartum women. BMI, body mass index; BNP, brain natriuretic peptide; BP, blood pressure; CBC, complete blood count; CTA, computed tomographic angiogram; EKG, electrocardiogram; HF, heart failure; HR, heart rate; MFM, maternal fetal medicine; NYHA, New York Heart Association; RR, relative risk; sat, saturation; TSH, thyroid stimulating hormone. (Afshan B. Hameed, Christine H. Morton, and Allana Moore. Improving Health Care Response to Cardiovascular Disease in Pregnancy and Postpartum Developed under contract #11-10006 with the California Department of Public Health, Maternal, Child and Adolescent Health Division. Published by the California Department of Public Health, 2017.)

underestimates the risk for many women who would otherwise qualify for closer follow-up monitoring. One study looking at the Framingham cardiovascular risk scores for postpartum women with hypertensive disorders in pregnancy found that scores were not higher in women with chronic hypertension complicated by superimposed preeclampsia or preeclampsia alone; however, women with gestational hypertension did have higher-risk scores than healthy controls.[17] In contrast, although another study found that women with chronic hypertension without superimposed preeclampsia had the highest median risk score (2.8%), this was not a high enough score to be stratified into a higher-risk category that may encourage more oversight for this population.[27] The initial calculator has been expanded to include 30-year and lifetime risk. With this change, about 50% of women with preeclampsia would be classified as being a lifetime high risk.[28]

Because 80% of all CVD is preventable through lifestyle modification and pharmacotherapy, identification of high-risk individuals is crucial.[29] Unfortunately, high-risk individuals are often not identified as such until much later in life when there is a potentially greater burden of disease.[29] If women could be identified following their first pregnancy complications for targeted screening, lifestyle modification, and early treatment, it may be possible to delay or decrease the chance of future clinical vascular or metabolic disease as well as the chance of developing complications in subsequent pregnancies.[30]

With the definition of hypertension changing to systolic blood pressure (SBP) greater than 130 mm Hg or diastolic blood pressure (DBP) greater than 90 mm Hg, 19% of women aged 20 to 44, prime childbearing years, will now carry the diagnosis of hypertension.[31] In addition, for women with a hypertensive disorder of pregnancy (eg, preeclampsia or gestational hypertension), between 56% and 67% are now classified as having hypertension at 6- to 12-months postpartum.[32] Given that more than half the deaths from coronary artery disease or stroke occur in people with a history of hypertension, cardiac care must orient itself toward acknowledging pregnancy as a crucial facet in predicting one's cardiovascular well-being.[33]

CARDIAC RISK BEYOND PREGNANCY

That age-adjusted death rates from coronary heart disease in women have declined since the 1980s is often attributed to a reduction in modifiable risk factors (cigarette smoking, diabetes, dyslipidemia, hypercholesterolemia, obesity, and low physical activity).[34,35] However, CVD still causes about 1 death per minute among women in the United States.[34] Research has shown that women meeting the AHA's definition of "ideal cardiovascular health" have greater longevity and reductions in short-term, intermediate-term, and lifetime risks for cardiovascular events.[36] This section discusses general goals of cardiac care as women approach menopause.

Although the total number of women dying from heart disease has decreased over the last several decades, cardiovascular death rates in women 35 to 54 years of age have started to increase again.[37] In large part, this is attributed to the worsening of modifiable risk factors in the general population, such as current cigarette smoking, diabetes, hypercholesterolemia, hypertension, obesity, physical inactivity, and unhealthy diet.[1,36] It is important to note that obesity alone largely contributes to mortality in patients with type 2 diabetes, which is primarily driven by the increased risk of stroke and myocardial infarction.[34,38] The AHA recommends actively managing these known risk factors.[36,37]

The AHA considers "relatively fixed" risk factors to be family history, increasing age, low socioeconomic or education status, and psychosocial stress.[1] Clearly, there are multiple risk factors that contribute to a woman's risk of cardiac disease. Traditionally, the Framingham Risk Score, a gender-specific algorithm that estimates the 10-year cardiovascular risk of an individual, has been used to stratify patients. However, the short-term focus (10 years) and use of limited end points (myocardial infarction and coronary heart disease death) do not guarantee that women deemed "low risk" do not have subclinical CVD.[39] In fact, a 2007 AHA panel determined that although a Framingham 10-year predicted risk greater than 20% could be used to identify a woman at high risk, a lower score was insufficient to ensure that she is at low risk.[37]

The AHA has also developed guidelines to determine an individual's cardiac risk. Their classifications incorporate the Framingham Risk Score as well as other known determinants of cardiac disease:

- At high risk: Documented CVD, diabetes mellitus, end-stage or chronic kidney disease, or a 10-year predicted risk for CVD greater than 10%
- At risk: Having greater than 1 major CVD risk factor, metabolic syndrome, subclinical coronary vascular disease (ie, coronary calcification), or poor exercise tolerance on the treadmill
- At optimal risk: Framingham Risk Score less than 10%, an absence of major CVD risk factors, and engagement in a healthy lifestyle

Since its initial publication in 2007, evidence has emerged to support the AHA's risk classification. Hsia and colleagues[40] evaluated 161,808 women aged 50 to 79 who were enrolled in the Women's Health Initiative. These women were followed for 7.8 years, after which they were assigned a risk based on the AHA guidelines. The rates of myocardial infarction and death were evaluated. The 2007 risk classification algorithm appropriately ordered all event rates in all groups, with a 7- to 20-fold difference in event rates between optimal-risk and high-risk women. Since its inception, the guideline was revised twice with the most recent version published in 2011.

In conjunction with its guidelines on cardiovascular risk, the AHA also publishes guidelines on blood pressure control. Given that hypertension can play a critical role in cardiovascular health, the two build on each other. As of the 2017 revision, an elevated blood pressure is SBP 120-129 mm Hg and a DBP <80 mm Hg. Hypertension is divided into stages, with stage 1 being SBP 130 to 139 mm Hg or DBP 80 to 89 mm Hg and stage 2 being SBP greater than 140 mm Hg or DBP greater than 90 mm Hg.[1,41]

Adults with elevated blood pressure or stage 1 hypertension who have an elevated 10-year CVD risk less than 10% should receive nonpharmacologic therapy and have a repeat blood pressure check in 3 to 6 months. Use of blood pressure–lowering medications is recommended for those with an average SBP of greater than 130 mm Hg or an average DBP of greater than 80 mm Hg. Weight loss is also recommended to reduce blood pressure.[36]

With the new criteria, care providers should anticipate that approximately one-fifth of women without a complication in pregnancy will be diagnosed with hypertension.[32] It is now being learned that in women who had pregnancy complicated by a hypertensive disorder, up to two-thirds, representing at least a doubling of the prevalence, will have diagnosable vascular disease.[32] Although lifestyle modification should still be the starting point for management, many more women may eventually require therapeutic interventions after the first 2 to 3 decades after pregnancy. There is a need for a longer-term approach to assessing cardiac risk rather than relying on stratifications of the past.

CARDIAC RISK IN POSTMENOPAUSAL WOMEN

As of July 2015, there are approximately 47.8 million people older than 65 years of age residing in the United States.[42] As of 2010, about 57% of this population are women, which is expected to hold steady over decades to come.[42] As previously discussed, there are many modifiable risk factors associated with future cardiac disease; however, advancing age is often an ignored major risk factor.[43,44] Incidence of diabetes, hypertension, coronary disease, and stroke steeply increases as people age. Although this can partially be attributed to accumulation of risk factors over time, age-associated changes in cardiovascular structure and function also play a role in the threshold, severity, and prognosis of CVD in the aging population.[43,45]

Both men and women experience the decline in vascular health; however, as women go through menopause, distinct physical changes occur that may make them further prone to CVD. It is well established that estrogen, and its derivatives, offers considerable cardioprotection.[46] In Dr Mary Jane Minkin's article, "Menopause: Hormones, Lifestyle, and Optimizing Aging," in this issue, she reviews menopause, hormone replacement therapy (HRT), and cardiovascular health. Although there is significant variation in circulating hormone levels in postmenopausal women, after menopause, estradiol levels are low and continue to decline with age.[47] Studies have found that although the absolute risk factor for CVD increases in midlife, menopause has a particularly adverse effect on lipid metabolism.[48] For example, the Healthy Women

Study (n = 372) found that there was a significant increase in LDL cholesterol and tri-glycerides levels during the perimenopause years, and that soon after menopause, women underwent their largest increase in blood pressure and fasting glucose.[48] Over the 5 years subjects were followed, there were marked changes in risk factors for CVD, such as SBP, pulse pressure, LDL and HDL cholesterol, triglycerides, fasting glucose, and body mass index.[48] Clearly, risk factor modification for premenopausal women may help mitigate development of CVD because age weakens the body's reserves.

Aside from maintaining a healthy diet and body weight, as discussed in Drs Eliza-beth A. Hoover and Judette M. Louis' article, "Optimizing Health: Weight, Exercise, and Nutrition in Pregnancy and Beyond," in this issue, cardioprotective measures are not complete without mention of HRT. In the late 1990s and early 2000s, several well-published trials suggested that HRT may cause coronary harm and increase a woman's risk for everything from stroke to breast cancer.[35,49,50] Widespread use of HRT was abruptly stopped. Concomitantly, with the cessation of HRT use, mortalities for women increased in 44% of US counties.[51] In those same counties, mortalities for men increased just 3%.[51] Although this may be attributable to many factors, given that reanalysis of the initial trial, as well as newer studies, has determined that use of HRT in younger women (ages 50–59 or within 10 years of menopause) actually decreases cor-onary disease and all-cause mortality, this change in practice may have had significant impact.[52–56] Today, data consistently note that HRT has a net benefit.[57–59] In Dr Mary Jane Minkin's article, "Menopause: Hormones, Lifestyle, and Optimizing Aging," in this issue, she presents a summary of both the historical literature and the North Amer-ica Menopause Society statements. Although there is a slightly increased risk of venous thrombosis in women on HRT, no other primary preventative strategy, aside from lifestyle modifications, has been found to be as beneficial.[59–61]

The distinct shift in cardiac risk that occurs once a woman enters menopause is largely ignored in routine screening guidelines. The USPSTF makes general sugges-tions for cardiovascular health, such as recommending blood pressure screening in adults over age 18 as well as advising a healthy diet and physical activity to overweight and obese adults.[62] The AHA/American College of Cardiology is more detailed, stating "it is reasonable to assess traditional ASCVD (atherosclerotic cardiovascular disease) risk factors every 4 to 6 years in adults 20 to 79 years of age who are free from ASCVD and to estimate 10-year ASCVD risk every 4 to 6 years in adults 40 to 79 years of age who are free from ASCVD."[63] Gender- and race-specific equations are currently avail-able to assess their cardiovascular risk more precisely. Although progress has been made, the standard of care still fails to recognize the intricacies of a woman's health cycle and the differing cardiovascular care she may need in each of these distinct periods.

SUMMARY

CVD remains an important cause of morbidity and mortality even in young women. Ed-ucation and awareness of the cardiovascular risk factors, including pregnancy compli-cations, are indicated to optimize outcomes by timely interventions. Initiatives, such as the WPSI, are a reminder to providers and patients alike that disease prevention must be focused on across a woman's lifespan.

REFERENCES

1. Lloyd-Jones DM, Morris PB, Ballantyne CM, et al. 2017 focused update of the 2016 ACC expert consensus decision pathway on the role of non-statin therapies

for LDL-cholesterol lowering in the management of atherosclerotic cardiovascular disease risk: a report of the American College of Cardiology Task Force on expert consensus decision. J Am Coll Cardiol 2017;70(14):1785–822.

2. Nemetz PN, Smith CY, Bailey KR, et al. Trends in coronary atherosclerosis: a tale of two population subgroups. Am J Med 2016;129(3):307–14.

3. Health Resources & Services Administration. Women's Preventive Services guidelines. U.S. Department of Health & Human Services. Available at: https://www.hrsa.gov/womens-guidelines/index.html.

4. Daniels SR, Greer FR. Lipid screening and cardiovascular health in childhood. Pediatrics 2008. https://doi.org/10.1542/peds.2008-1349.

5. Webber LS, Osganian V, Luepker RV, et al. Cardiovascular risk factors among third grade children in four regions of the united states: the catch study. Am J Epidemiol 1995. https://doi.org/10.1093/oxfordjournals.aje.a117445.

6. Haney EM, Huffman LH, Bougatsos C, et al. Screening and treatment for lipid disorders in children and adolescents: systematic evidence review for the US Preventive Services Task Force. Pediatrics 2007. https://doi.org/10.1542/peds.2006-1801.

7. Boney CM, Verma A, Tucker R, et al. American Academy of Pediatrics. National Cholesterol Education Program: report of the expert panel on blood cholesterol levels in children and adolescents. Pediatrics 1992. https://doi.org/10.1542/peds.103.6.1175.

8. Dennison BA, Jenkins PL, Pearson TA. Challenges to implementing the current pediatric cholesterol screening guidelines into practice. Pediatrics 1994. https://doi.org/10.3138/jsp.47.2.105.

9. Williams RR, Hunt SC, Barlow GK, et al. Prevention of familial cardiovascular disease by screening for family history and lipids in youths. Clin Chem 1992.

10. Rifai N, Neufeld E, Ahlstrom P, et al. Failure of current guidelines for cholesterol screening in urban African-American adolescents. Pediatrics 1996. https://doi.org/10.1002/cyto.a.20671.

11. Kirk S, Zeller M, Claytor R, et al. The relationship of health outcomes to improvement in BMI in children and adolescents. Obes Res 2005. https://doi.org/10.1038/oby.2005.101.

12. AHA. 2015-2020 dietary guidelines for Americans. Washington, DC: Health.gov; 2016. https://doi.org/10.1097/NT.0b013e31826c50af.

13. Gidding SS, Dennison BA, Birch LL, et al. Dietary recommendations for children and adolescents: a guide for practitioners. Pediatrics 2006. https://doi.org/10.1542/peds.2005-2374.

14. Mayer-Davis EJ, Lawrence JM, Dabelea D, et al. Incidence trends of type 1 and type 2 diabetes among youths, 2002–2012. N Engl J Med 2017. https://doi.org/10.1056/NEJMoa1610187.

15. Anyaegbu EI, Dharnidharka VR. Hypertension in the teenager. Pediatr Clin North Am 2014. https://doi.org/10.1016/j.pcl.2013.09.011.

16. Saade GR. Pregnancy as a window to future health. Obstet Gynecol 2009. https://doi.org/10.1097/AOG.0b013e3181bf5588.

17. Escouto DC, Green A, Kurlak L, et al. Postpartum evaluation of cardiovascular disease risk for women with pregnancies complicated by hypertension. Pregnancy Hypertens 2018;13:218–24.

18. Irgens HU, Reisaeter L, Irgens LM, et al. Long term mortality of mothers and fathers after pre-eclampsia: population based cohort study. BMJ 2001. https://doi.org/10.1136/bmj.323.7323.1213.

19. Bellamy L, Casas JP, Hingorani AD, et al. Pre-eclampsia and risk of cardiovascular disease and cancer in later life: systematic review and meta-analysis. Br Med J 2007. https://doi.org/10.1136/bmj.39335.385301.BE.

20. Cirillo PM, Cohn BA. Pregnancy complications and cardiovascular disease death 50-year follow-up of the child health and development studies pregnancy cohort. Circulation 2015. https://doi.org/10.1161/CIRCULATIONAHA.113.003901.

21. Garovic VD, Hayman SR. Hypertension in pregnancy: an emerging risk factor for cardiovascular disease. Nat Clin Pract Nephrol 2007. https://doi.org/10.1038/ncpneph0623.

22. Smith GN. The maternal health clinic: improving women's cardiovascular health. Semin Perinatol 2015;39(4):316–9.

23. Murphy MSQ, Smith GN. Pre-eclampsia and cardiovascular disease risk assessment in women. Am J Perinatol 2016;33(8):723–31.

24. Cusimano MC, Pudwell J, Roddy M, et al. The maternal health clinic: an initiative for cardiovascular risk identification in women with pregnancy-related complications. Am J Obstet Gynecol 2014. https://doi.org/10.1016/j.ajog.2013.12.001.

25. Disease C, Pregnancy IN, Toolkit P. Cardiovascular disease assessment in pregnant. 2017;(November):7-12.

26. Brown MC, Best KE, Pearce MS, et al. Cardiovascular disease risk in women with pre-eclampsia: systematic review and meta-analysis. Eur J Epidemiol 2013. https://doi.org/10.1007/s10654-013-9762-6.

27. Brown MA, Lindheimer MD, De Swiet M, et al. The classification and diagnosis of the hypertensive disorders of pregnancy: statement from the International Society for the Study of Hypertension in Pregnancy (ISSHP). Hypertens Pregnancy 2001. https://doi.org/10.1081/PRG-100104165.

28. Smith GN, Pudwell J, Walker M, et al. Ten-year, thirty-year, and lifetime cardiovascular disease risk estimates following a pregnancy complicated by preeclampsia. J Obstet Gynaecol Can 2012. https://doi.org/10.1016/S1701-2163(16)35381-6.

29. Smith GN, Walker MC, Liu A, et al. A history of preeclampsia identifies women who have underlying cardiovascular risk factors. Am J Obstet Gynecol 2009. https://doi.org/10.1016/j.ajog.2008.06.035.

30. Rich-Edwards JW, McElrath TF, Karumanchi SA, et al. Breathing life into the life-course approach: pregnancy history and cardiovascular disease in women. Hypertension 2010. https://doi.org/10.1161/HYPERTENSIONAHA.110.156810.

31. Whelton PK, Carey RM, Aronow WS, et al. 2017 ACC/AHA/AAPA/ABC/ACPM/AGS/APhA/ASH/ASPC/NMA/PCNA guideline for the prevention, detection, evaluation, and management of high blood pressure in adults: a report of the American College of Cardiology/American Heart Association Task Force on clinical practice guidelines. Hypertension 2018. https://doi.org/10.1161/HYP.0000000000000065.

32. Smith G, Pudwell J, Saade G. Impact of the new American hypertension guidelines on the prevalence of postpartum hypertension. Am J Perinatol 2018;2–4. https://doi.org/10.1055/s-0038-1669441.

33. Ford ES. Trends in mortality from all causes and cardiovascular disease among hypertensive and nonhypertensive adults in the United States. Circulation 2011. https://doi.org/10.1161/CIRCULATIONAHA.110.005645.

34. Roger VL, Go AS, Lloyd-Jones DM, et al. Heart disease and stroke statistics—2011 update: a report from the American Heart Association. Circulation 2011. https://doi.org/10.1161/CIR.0b013e3182009701.

35. Writing Group for the Women's Health Initiative Investigators. Risks and benefits of estrogen plus progestin in healthy postmenopausal women: principal results

from the Women's Health Initiative randomized controlled trial. JAMA 2002. https://doi.org/10.1001/jama.288.3.321.

36. Lloyd-Jones DM, Hong Y, Labarthe D, et al. Defining and setting national goals for cardiovascular health promotion and disease reduction: the American Heart Association's strategic impact goal through 2020 and beyond. Circulation 2010. https://doi.org/10.1161/CIRCULATIONAHA.109.192703.

37. Mosca L, Benjamin EJ, Berra K, et al. Effectiveness-based guidelines for the prevention of cardiovascular disease in women—2011 update: a guideline from the American Heart Association. Circulation 2011;123(11):1243–62.

38. Preis SR, Hwang SJ, Coady S, et al. Trends in all cause and cardiovascular disease mortality among women and men with and without diabetes mellitus in the Framingham Heart Study, 1950 to 2005. Circulation 2009. https://doi.org/10.1161/CIRCULATIONAHA.108.829176.

39. Fuster V, Rydén LE, Cannom DS, et al. 2011 ACCF/AHA/HRS focused updates incorporated into the ACC/AHA/ESC 2006 guidelines for the management of patients with atrial fibrillation: a report of the American College of Cardiology Foundation/American Heart Association Task Force on practice guidel. J Am Coll Cardiol 2011. https://doi.org/10.1016/j.jacc.2010.09.013.

40. Hsia J, Rodabough RJ, Manson JE, et al. Evaluation of the American Heart Association cardiovascular disease prevention guideline for women. Circ Cardiovasc Qual Outcomes 2010. https://doi.org/10.1161/CIRCOUTCOMES.108.842385.

41. McManus RJ, Mant J. Hypertension: new US blood-pressure guidelines—who asked the patients? Nat Rev Cardiol 2018;15(3):137–8.

42. Vincent GK, Velkoff VA. The next four decades the older population in the United States: 2010 to 2050. Curr Popul Reports 2010;2011:P25–1138. U.S. Census Bureau, Washington, DC.

43. Lakatta EG, Levy D. Arterial and cardiac aging: major shareholders in cardiovascular disease enterprises: part I: aging arteries: a "set up" for vascular disease. Circulation 2003. https://doi.org/10.1161/01.CIR.0000048892.83521.58.

44. Najjar SS, Scuteri A, Lakatta EG. Arterial aging: is it an immutable cardiovascular risk factor? Hypertension 2005. https://doi.org/10.1161/01.HYP.0000177474.06749.98.

45. Fleg JL, O'Connor F, Gerstenblith G, et al. Impact of age on the cardiovascular response to dynamic upright exercise in healthy men and women. J Appl Physiol (1985) 1995. https://doi.org/10.1152/jappl.1995.78.3.890.

46. Subbiah MT. Mechanisms of cardioprotection by estrogens. Proc Soc Exp Biol Med 1998;217(1):23–9.

47. Longcope C, Franz C, Morello C, et al. Steroid and gonadotropin levels in women during the peri-menopausal years. Maturitas 1986. https://doi.org/10.1016/0378-5122(86)90025-3.

48. Matthews KA, Kuller LH, Sutton-Tyrrell K, et al. Changes in cardiovascular risk factors during the perimenopause and postmenopause and carotid artery atherosclerosis in healthy women. Stroke 2001;32(5):1104–11.

49. Hulley S, Grady D, Bush T, et al. Randomized trial of estrogen plus progestin for secondary prevention of coronary heart disease in postmenopausal women. J Am Med Assoc 1998. https://doi.org/10.1001/jama.280.7.605.

50. Clarke SC, Kelleher J, Lloyd-Jones H, et al. A study of hormone replacement therapy in postmenopausal women with ischaemic heart disease: the Papworth HRT Atherosclerosis Study. BJOG 2002. https://doi.org/10.1111/j.1471-0528.2002.01544.x.

51. Kindig DA, Cheng ER. Even as mortality fell in most US counties, female mortality nonetheless rose in 42.8 percent of counties from 1992 to 2006. Health Aff 2013. https://doi.org/10.1377/hlthaff.2011.0892.
52. Stampfer MJ, Colditz GA. Estrogen replacement therapy and coronary heart disease: a quantitative assessment of the epidemiologic evidence. Prev Med (Baltim) 1991. https://doi.org/10.1016/0091-7435(91)90006-P.
53. Grodstein F, Stampfer MJ, Colditz GA, et al. Postmenopausal hormone therapy and mortality. N Engl J Med 1997. https://doi.org/10.1056/NEJM199706193362501.
54. Yaffe K, Sawaya G, Lieberburg I, et al. Estrogen therapy in postmenopausal women: effects on cognitive function and dementia. J Am Med Assoc 1998. https://doi.org/10.1001/jama.279.9.688.
55. Henderson BE, Paganini Hill A, Ross RK. Decreased mortality in users of estrogen replacement therapy. Arch Intern Med 1991. https://doi.org/10.1001/archinte.1991.00400010095012.
56. Grady D, Rubin SM, Petitti DB, et al. Hormone therapy to prevent disease and prolong life in postmenopausal women. Ann Intern Med 1992. https://doi.org/10.7326/0003-4819-117-12-1016.
57. Manson JAE, Chlebowski RT, Stefanick ML, et al. Menopausal hormone therapy and health outcomes during the intervention and extended poststopping phases of the women's health initiative randomized trials. Obstet Gynecol Surv 2014. https://doi.org/10.1097/01.ogx.0000444679.66386.38.
58. Schierbeck LL, Rejnmark L, Tofteng CL, et al. Effect of hormone replacement therapy on cardiovascular events in recently postmenopausal women: randomised trial. BMJ 2012. https://doi.org/10.1136/bmj.e6409.
59. Lobo RA, Pickar JH, Stevenson JC, et al. Back to the future: hormone replacement therapy as part of a prevention strategy for women at the onset of menopause. Atherosclerosis 2016;254:282–90.
60. Bergendal A, Kieler H, Sundström A, et al. Risk of venous thromboembolism associated with local and systemic use of hormone therapy in peri- and postmenopausal women and in relation to type and route of administration. Menopause 2016. https://doi.org/10.1097/GME.0000000000000611.
61. Lobo RA, Davis SR, De Villiers TJ, et al. Prevention of diseases after menopause. Climacteric 2014. https://doi.org/10.3109/13697137.2014.933411.
62. Services USP, Force T. USPSTF A and B recommendations. Search; 2010.
63. Goff DC, Lloyd-jones DM, Bennett G, et al. Reply: 2013 ACC/AHA guideline on the assessment of cardiovascular risk. J Am Coll Cardiol 2014;63(25):2886.

Section 3: Post Maturity

Pelvic Floor Disorders

Meadow Maze Good, DO, FACOG[a],*, Ellen R. Solomon, MD, FACOG[b]

KEYWORDS

- Pelvic floor disorders • Urinary incontinence • Pelvic organ prolapse

KEY POINTS

- Pelvic floor disorders, including urinary incontinence and pelvic organ prolapse, are common and may negatively affect a woman's self-image and quality of life at any age.
- Maintaining a healthy lifestyle (eating well, exercising, and avoiding constipation), is essential for optimal bladder health and function.
- Women's health care providers should be prepared to routinely ask and discuss the most common issues affecting those with pelvic floor issues and offer urinary incontinence and pelvic organ prolapse treatment options in a stepwise fashion.

Genitourinary health is an essential topic that should be addressed by every health care provider when caring for women throughout her lifetime. Pelvic floor disorders (PFDs), including urinary incontinence and pelvic organ prolapse (POP), may affect women of any age and negatively affect a woman's self-image and quality of life. Unfortunately, in many societies, these conditions may lead to stigmatization; in turn, women may delay care or not seek help. Studies have shown that treating women with incontinence or prolapse can positively influence their quality of life and sexual satisfaction. Overall, these disorders affecting women of all ages are underrecognized and undertreated.

PELVIC FLOOR DISORDERS

It is estimated that women have a 1 in 4 lifetime risk of experiencing a PFD. With multifactorial etiologic factors, damage to the pelvic floor may lead to urinary incontinence, anal incontinence, POP, and sexual dysfunction. Increasing age, weight, parity, and a history of hysterectomy are all risk factors for PFDs, with approximately

Disclosure Statement: The authors have nothing to disclose.
[a] Department of Obstetrics and Gynecology, Division of Female Pelvic Medicine & Reconstructive Surgery, University of Florida College of Medicine Jacksonville, Jacksonville, FL, USA;
[b] Obstetrics and Gynecology, Division of Female Pelvic Surgery, University of Massachusetts–Baystate Medical Center, 759 Chestnut Street, Springfield, MA 01199, USA
* Corresponding author. Department of Obstetrics and Gynecology, Division of FPMRS, 653-1 West 8th Street, LRC 3rd Floor, Jacksonville, FL 32209.
E-mail address: Meadow.Good@jax.ufl.edu
; @meadowgood (M.M.G.)

Obstet Gynecol Clin N Am 46 (2019) 527–540
https://doi.org/10.1016/j.ogc.2019.04.010
0889-8545/19/Published by Elsevier Inc.
obgyn.theclinics.com

17% of women being affected in their lifetime. As women age the prevalence increases, with greater than 40% of women older than 40 years old experiencing urinary incontinence.[1] Additionally, POP is common, with 30% to 76% of women presenting for routine gynecologic care with loss of pelvic floor support on exam, leading to 300,000 surgeries per year in the United States alone.[2] Risk factors for developing a PFD include increasing age (menopausal status), prior hysterectomy, vaginal birth, obesity, smoking, and inheriting a connective tissue disorder. The Women's Preventive Services Initiative recommends screening all women annually, regardless of age or parity, for urinary incontinence. Screening should assess whether women experience incontinence or prolapse symptoms, and whether it affects their quality of life. Useful validated questionnaires are available to help assess whether a woman is experiencing bothersome urinary incontinence or prolapse symptoms. Many women silently suffer with PFDs, incorrectly believing that incontinence and prolapse are a normal consequence of aging. Women's health care providers have the ability to screen women for PFDs who may be silently suffering and help them find appropriately trained physicians to care for these issues.

Female Pelvic Medicine and Reconstructive Surgery (FPMRS) is a combined board-certified subspecialty of both Obstetrics and Gynecology, and Urology accredited through the American Board of Medical Specialties. Urogynecology is the term ob-gyns use to describe an ob-gyn who has FPMRS subspecialty training. Physicians graduating from these fellowships take both written and oral boards on the subject matter, and have specialized training for treating PFDs. A qualified physician may be found via the Voices for Pelvic Floor Disorders Web site (www.voicesforpfd.org), a valuable resource for both patients and physicians, and maintained by the American Urogynecologic Society. Although most treatments for PFDs are considered elective, a woman's symptoms may be embarrassing, debilitating, and limit her ability to lead a normal life. Fortunately, there are many treatment options for women suffering with PFDs and FPMRS specialists are readily available to educate women with a stepwise approach, starting with the most conservative options first.

Multidisciplinary team-approached care for a woman with pelvic floor conditions may be helpful. Such teams include nurse care coordinators, pelvic floor physical therapists, urogynecologists, colorectal surgeons, urologists, and geriatricians. Having this team in place to support the patient may facilitate the stepwise approach and allow the patient to feel comfortable with the needed level of care. Although little data exist regarding superior outcomes with this approach, it is promising.[3]

EVALUATION AND DIAGNOSIS

Diagnosis should involve a thorough background history and physical examination. Developing a routine of asking a patient questions regarding incontinence and prolapse symptoms may be helpful in identifying patients who have pelvic floor issues. Consider including questions such as

1. Do you feel you urinate more than normal during the day or night?
2. Do you have bladder accidents when you cough, laugh, exercise, or when trying to get to the toilet to urinate?
3. Do you feel a bulge, ball, or pressure in the vagina?

Because patients will not volunteer embarrassing information, it is important ask. Using a review of a symptoms chart or a short validated questionnaire in the intake form may be the first step in getting the patient the resources she needs to improve her life. Patients may fill out standardized severity questionnaires to determine the level of bother that the patient is experiencing and to estimate what the examination may present. For pelvic floor symptoms, using the Pelvic Floor Disability Index-20 may be most helpful.

Detailed medical history includes interviewing for other symptoms of medical conditions that may cause urinary incontinence as part of their disease process. For example, it is important to ask about diabetes, multiple sclerosis, thyroid disease, prior cerebrovascular injury, prior spinal cord injury, back pain, prior back injuries, and urologic conditions (recurrent urinary tract infections, kidney stones, and gross hematuria).

Commonly prescribed medications may also interfere with the bladder's ability to function normally. Muscle relaxants, narcotics, alpha-blocking agents, and selective antihypertensive drugs (calcium-channel blockers and methyldopa) may exacerbate urethral smooth and skeletal muscle relaxation, causing stress urinary incontinence (SUI). Antihistamine and anticholinergic effects may be additive and lead to urinary hesitancy and retention. Decongestants and some diet medication have alpha-adrenergic effects and may cause urinary retention by preventing the urethral sphincter's normal function.

A physical examination should include a detailed genitourinary and pelvic floor examination to help find any anatomic causes for the patient's symptoms. The examination should include

- A visual inspection of the genital area
- Evaluation of nerve conduction
- Observation of urethral hypermobility with cough and/or Valsalva stress test
- Urethral palpation for abnormalities
- A standardized vaginal examination using a prolapse grading system
- Evaluation of the levator ani for tone and strength
- A bimanual examination to evaluate the uterus, cervix, and adnexa.

Laboratory tests, including a urinalysis with microscopy and urine culture, are important for thorough evaluation of PFDs to rule out infection and symptomatic microscopic hematuria. Additionally, obtaining an assessment of the postvoid residual volume ensures adequate emptying and is necessary before treatment. This can be done via ultrasound or an in-and-out catheter after voiding.

NORMAL BLADDER HEALTH

The bladder is a sensitive organ. In general, recommending a healthy lifestyle is essential for optimal health, including the bladder. Eating well, exercising, and avoiding constipation may all play a role in how the bladder functions. A patient should normally urinate 7 or fewer times per day with a volume of approximately 300 to 700 mL and not wake to void at night. Normal postvoid residuals should be less than 100 to 150 mL.[4]

Common medical conditions and medications may contribute to urinary issues. It is important to recognize symptoms that may be urinary in nature but could point to an underlying medical condition. Diabetes, hypothyroidism, constipation, and genitourinary syndrome of menopause (formerly known as atrophic vaginitis) may lead to urinary symptoms; therefore, it is important to evaluate for these conditions if indicated before medically treating an overactive bladder (OAB).

Avoiding constipation is essential to normal bladder function. When the rectum is full of stool, it may cause the patient to feel an increased need to urinate frequently or urgently. Having a high-fiber diet may improve bowel and bladder function. Using a stool or "Squatty Potty" in front of the toilet to put one's feet on while defecating can aid in achieving a natural squatting position and help empty the rectum.

Discuss hydration habits with patients. Have them drink enough liquids (water) each day. In general, it may be helpful to advise them to drink water with meals and then drink one 16 oz (sports-sized bottle) of water throughout the day to stay hydrated. Water is the best liquid for the bladder. If there is a problem with incontinence, do not limit fluid intake because this can cause concentrated urine, which may further irritate the bladder. It is also important to not have patients force drink; they should listen to their thirst mechanism.

Discussing good toileting habits can improve both bladder and bowel function. Have patient's sit on the toilet seat with their feet on a stool or the ground and relax when emptying the bladder and bowels. Advise them not to strain and let the bladder do the work. Women should not hover above the toilet because this contracts the pelvic floor, in direct opposition to the relaxation needed to void properly. Have women empty their bladder no more or less than every 3 to 4 hours. If there is an urgent need to go to the bathroom, advise them not to wait until it becomes an emergency.

The bladder is a sensitive organ. Some foods and beverages, increasing the incontinence symptoms as may increase bladder activity, increasing irritative voiding or incontinence symptoms. Limiting or eliminating the following may help:

- Alcohol
- Caffeine (cola, tea, and coffee)
- Acidic foods or beverages, including citrus and tomatoes
- Sugar or honey
- Artificial sweeteners, such as aspartame
- Spicy foods
- Cigarettes.

Symptoms that a patient may experience that would warrant further workup and necessitate a referral to a urogynecologist include:

- Difficulty starting the stream of urination
- Feelings of incomplete bladder emptying
- Needing to urinate frequently or urgently (OAB)
- Pain with urination
- Foul smelling or cloudy urine
- Urinating at night (nocturia)
- Leaking of urine
- Bladder pain
- Blood in the urine
- Dribbling after urination

URINARY INCONTINENCE

Urinary incontinence is the unintentional leakage of urine. The most important consideration is the degree of bother a woman has accompanying the leaking. Urinary incontinence, per the International Continence Society, is both a symptom, defined as "complaint of involuntary leakage of urine," and a sign, defined as the "observation of involuntary loss of urine on examination."

There are 2 main subtypes of urinary incontinence: urgency and stress. Urgency incontinence occurs with a sudden overwhelming desire to void, whereas stress incontinence occurs with physical exertion. OAB, a broader term, includes urinary urgency and/or frequency with or without incontinence, and nocturia. Urinary frequency is defined as voiding more than 7 times per day and voiding 1 or more times at night. Mixed incontinence is the term used when a woman has both stress and urgency types of incontinence. Although it is never normal to leak urine involuntarily, the changes to the urinary tract as women age may predispose voiding issues. Other risk factors for developing urinary incontinence include genetics, race, multiparity, obesity, smoking, and increased body mass index. As described previously, having healthy habits, including food and beverage choices, and toileting (urinary and defecatory), can help improve or resolve some urinary issues. A stepwise approach to treatment may be most useful in patients with urinary complaints that include OAB and urgency or stress urinary incontinence (**Figs. 1** and **2**). Starting with the most conservative, least invasive options, patients should be educated about all treatment choices and encouraged to start with the basics and work up to procedural interventions.

URGENCY URINARY INCONTINENCE

Urgency urinary incontinence, per the International Continence Society, is defined as the "complaint of involuntary loss of urine associated with urgency." Common triggers to this bothersome issue include putting keys in the door, washing hands, or running the water. The main mechanism of urinary urgency may be caused by the bladder contracting at inappropriate times and the patient lacking control with the perceived contraction. Additionally, bladder hypersensitivity and poor bladder compliance may be factors. Contraction of the detrusor may or may not be seen during urodynamic evaluation; however, this does not mean that it does not play a role in the mechanism of the incontinence.

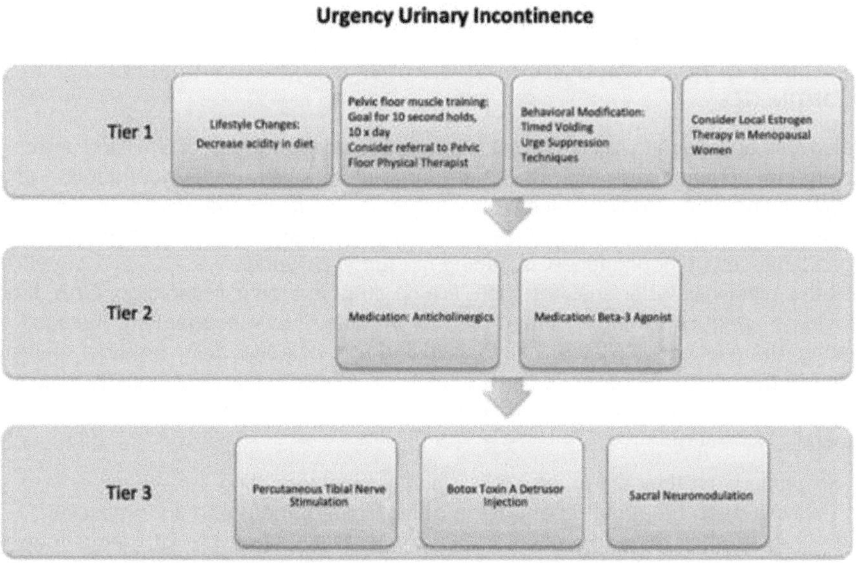

Urgency Urinary Incontinence

Tier 1	Lifestyle Changes: Decrease acidity in diet	Pelvic floor muscle training: Goal for 10 second holds, 10 x day Consider referral to Pelvic Floor Physical Therapist	Behavioral Modification: Timed Voiding Urge Suppression Techniques	Consider Local Estrogen Therapy in Menopausal Women

Tier 2	Medication: Anticholinergics	Medication: Beta-3 Agonist

Tier 3	Percutaneous Tibial Nerve Stimulation	Botox Toxin A Detrusor Injection	Sacral Neuromodulation

Fig. 1. Stepwise management of Urgency Urinary Incontinence.

STRESS URINARY INCONTINENCE

As defined by the International Continence Society, SUI is the "Complaint of involuntary loss of urine on effort or physical exertion including sporting activities, or on sneezing or coughing." There are 2 known mechanisms for causing SUI: urethral hypermobility from pelvic floor weakness and weakness of the urethral sphincter itself. The lifetime risk for undergoing surgery to address SUI is 20.5%.[1] Many options exist for treatment of this condition.

Stress Urinary Incontinence

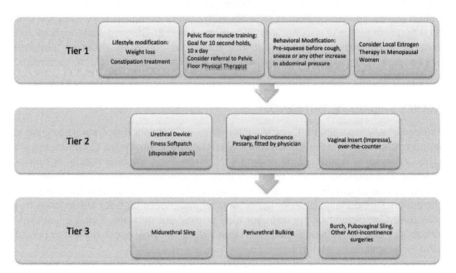

Fig. 2. Stepwise management of Stress Urinary Incontinence.

TREATMENT OPTIONS FOR OVERACTIVE BLADDER OR URGENCY URINARY INCONTINENCE

A stepwise approach to management is advised for the treatment of OAB and urgency urinary incontinence (see **Fig. 1**). Patient education is key. Patient completion of a 3-day voiding diary, followed by the provider reviewing it with the patient, is beneficial for the patient and clinician to establish behavioral patterns and to rule out other organic causes of incontinence, including nocturnal polyuria.

At the initial visit, after ensuring there are no other anatomic reasons for OAB, time should be spent reviewing common bladder irritants, fluid management, medication oversight and effects, toileting habits, and the role of pelvic floor physical therapy (PT) with the use of the pelvic floor muscles to suppress the urge. Various techniques are used to encourage patients who experience sudden uncontrollable urges, which generally consist of

1. Stopping what they are doing and staying in place or sitting
2. Taking a deep breath and performing quick flicks of the pelvic floor muscles
3. Distracting their mind (eg, count to 100 by 7s, make a grocery list, sing a song in their head); should be practiced and perfected so that it can be used as needed.

Weight reduction in women who are overweight or obese can dramatically reduce urinary symptoms and affect quality of life. One study showed reduction in weight by 3% to 5% may result in about a 50% reduction in incontinence episodes.[3] Pelvic floor muscle therapy or, in some cases, pelvic floor PT can improve function and control over the pelvic floor muscles, thus leading to better control of the experienced urinary urge.

After ensuring the bowels are working without constipation or diarrhea and the patient has been taught pelvic floor muscle exercises or referred to pelvic floor physical therapy, medication is usually the next step. In general, medication should be expected to reduce the number of urgency urine incontinence (UUI) episodes by 1 to 3 per day. One study comparing anticholinergics to onabotulinumtoxin A showed a similar reduction in UUI episodes by 3 per day in both groups.[5] Anticholinergics and beta-3 agonists are the 2 types of drugs that are available to treat OAB or UUI. More than 86 good quality trials exist showing there are several efficacious drugs to treat OAB. The 2 most studied drugs are oxybutynin and tolterodine, with similar efficacy and side effects. Dry mouth is a consistent reason for discontinuation and it may be better if long-acting preparations are used. Solifenacin may have better efficacy and better side effects. Unlike other anticholinergics, trospium is a larger sized molecule (quaternary amine) and, theoretically, should not cross the blood–brain barrier. Many recent concerns have been published regarding the use of anticholinergics in the elderly because there may be additive cognitive effects.[6] Caution should be exercised in the use of these medications in the elderly; however, avoidance or discontinuation may deprive patients of the benefits of improved quality of life from treatment for which alternative managements currently remain limited.

A beta-3 agonist is available, mirabegron, which has shown better tolerability because it should not have anticholinergic side effects. This class is not advised in those with uncontrolled cardiac issues (uncontrolled hypertension) and blood pressure should be monitored after starting this medication.

If a patient has failed or cannot tolerate 2 or more drugs, third-line options are available. These options include

1. Onabotulinumtoxin toxin A injections into the detrusor muscle
2. Percutaneous tibial nerve stimulation (PTNS)
3. Sacral neuromodulation

In a recent study comparing the cost-effectiveness of third-line treatments, onabotulinumtoxin toxin A injection was the most cost-effective option for patients with refractory OAB.[7]

TREATMENT OPTIONS FOR STRESS URINARY INCONTINENCE

Patients should be educated about all treatment options for SUI and encouraged to start with conservative management and work up to procedural interventions. A stepwise approach to treatment is advised (see **Fig. 2**). Behavioral modifications may improve SUI symptoms. As previously mentioned, losing 5% to 10% of weight may reduce SUI symptoms. Referring a patient to pelvic floor PT for pelvic floor muscle exercises and professional guidance may also be a suitable treatment option. A randomized controlled trial comparing pessary use with behavioral therapy or combined therapy showed that behavioral therapy resulted in greater patient satisfaction and fewer short-term symptoms; however, this did not persist at the 1-year point.[8]

A patient may try absorbance devices, including special undergarments and pads. Devices are available over-the-counter to reduce stress leakage, such as Finess Softpatch disposable occlusive patches, which temporarily cover the urethra, and Poise Impressa vaginal inserts. In the urogynecologist's office, many types of incontinence pessaries are available. Most commonly, a ring or dish with a continence knob may be placed in the vagina with the knob facing anteriorly to provide urethral support (**Fig. 3**). This is a great option that should be explored for most women. As shown in a multicenter study, 92% of women are successfully fitted for a continence pessary and most do not need to try more than 2 pessaries to find a comfortable fit.[9]

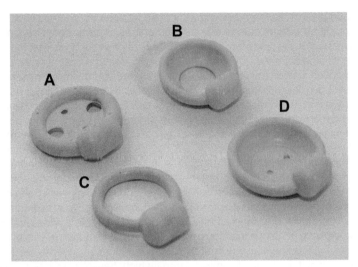

Fig. 3. Stress urinary incontinence pessaries.

Last options are surgical procedures that may immediately and drastically improve a patient's life. The gold standard anti-SUI procedure is the midurethral sling. With greater than 80% efficacy in curing SUI, it is difficult not to want to offer this option first. Educating the patient on all of the options and offering a step-wise approach will help to maximize patient satisfaction. Urethral bulking is an option with 60% to 70% improvement in symptoms and is a great choice for someone who is not a good surgical candidate in the operating room because it can be performed in the office. The patient should be informed that additional injections may be necessary in the future.

PELVIC ORGAN PROLAPSE

POP is a common and often distressing condition that women may experience. Because of the embarrassing nature of prolapse and its subsequent symptoms, many patients may not bring up concerns to their physicians and/or believe that prolapse symptoms are a normal condition that coincides with aging.

Patients with prolapse may present with

- A feeling of bulge at the perineum
- Feeling like they are sitting on a ball, egg, or meatball
- Low back pain
- Difficulty voiding or defecating
- Need to place a hand or fingers in the vagina to urinate or defecate
- Need to place hand or fingers on the perineum or around the anus to defecate.

Definitions

POP is defined as "a descent of the anterior or posterior vaginal wall, or descent of the uterus (or the vaginal vault after hysterectomy)."[10] Symptomatic POP is a common condition that occurs when there is a herniation of the pelvic organs through the vagina. Patients with symptomatic POP may present with a feeling of sitting on a ball or egg. They may notice tissue protruding through the vagina and they may have difficulty voiding or passing stool because of the noticeable bulge. Some patients may place their fingers in the vagina to empty their bladder or rectum, or press on the perineum to pass stool; this is called splinting. Prolapse may lead to urinary and defecatory dysfunction. A herniation of the most superior aspect of the vagina, which can include the vaginal cuff or the cervix, is called apical prolapse. Herniation of the anterior vaginal wall is sometimes referred to as a cystocele or dropped bladder but should be referred to as anterior vaginal wall prolapse. Herniation of the posterior wall is called a rectocele or posterior vaginal prolapse. The small bowel may also herniate through the vagina and this is called an enterocele. Defining the amount of prolapse can be performed using 2 different types of scales: the Badin-Walker scale, graded from 0 to 4, and the POP Quantification (POP-Q) scale, staged from 0 to 4. For purposes of description in this article, POP-Q is used to describe prolapse. The most important symptom is the degree of bother the patient is experiencing with the condition.

The POP-Q measures 9 different points in the vagina, is a standardized method to measure prolapse, and provides objective data for the examiner that can be used both clinically and experimentally. The hymen is used as the fixed point of measurement and is defined as 0. Points are measured from the hymen and may be negative (superior to the hymen) or positive (inferior to the hymen). The genital hiatus is measured from mid urethra to the hymen. The perineal body is measured from the hymen to mid anus. The total vaginal length (TVL) is measured from the hymen to the cervix or vaginal cuff. Point Aa is measured in the midline of the anterior vaginal wall, 3 cm from the urethral meatus, and can measure from −3 to +3 cm. Point Ap is the most dependent portion of any part of the anterior vaginal wall between point Aa and the vaginal cuff or anterior fornix. For the posterior vagina, point Ba is measured 3 cm from the hymenal ring in the midline of the posterior vagina, and point Bp is measured 3 cm from point Ba and is the most dependent portion of the prolapse to the posterior fourchette. There are 5 stages of prolapse measured from 0 to 4. **Fig. 4** shows the specific staging.[11]

To understand how and why prolapse occurs and what structures are injured, it is helpful to the 3 levels of the DeLancey levels of pelvic support.[12] Level 1 includes the cardinal-uterosacral ligament complex, which is where the apex of the uterus and vaginal vault are attached to the bony sacrum. Uterine and apical prolapse will occur when this level of support is damaged or weakened. Level 2 includes the levator ani muscles and the arcus tendinous fascia pelvis provides support for the midvagina, as well as to parts of the anterior and posterior vaginal walls. Level 3 includes the urogenital diaphragm and the perineal body, which supports the lower vagina. These definitions will be used in later discussion of surgical correction.

Evaluation and Diagnosis

As previously mentioned, a thorough patient history and a physical need to be performed to evaluate prolapse. Before performing the history and physical, any relevant standardized questionnaires may be used to assess the degree of bother. Questions regarding bulge and pressure, as well as splinting or having to push on vagina or rectum to void or defecate, are highly specific to prolapse and, if positive, will most likely indicate an objective prolapse. Other important histories include obstetric and gynecologic history, including number of pregnancies, route of delivery, and age at menopause. Prolapse often is from a genetic component and often patients may be able to give a family history of a connective tissue disorder or their mothers or aunts who have had a hysterectomy for prolapse.

As previously discussed, a thorough investigation of bladder issues is also obtained during the history and physical portion. A cystocele or rectocele may cause difficulty emptying the bladder because of obstructing symptoms. Often, patients with bladder

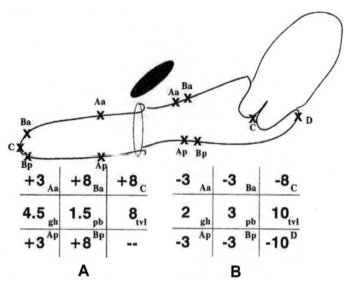

Fig. 4. Stage of prolapse: stage 0 (points Aa, Ba, Ap, Bp at −3 cm and C or D < TVL −2 cm), stage I (leading edge of prolapse <−1 cm and not stage 0), stage II (leading edge of prolapse >−1 cm but <+1 cm), stage III (leading edge of prolapse >+1 cm but < TVL-2 cm), and stage IV (leading edge of prolapse > TVL −2 cm). (A) Grid and line diagram of complete eversion of vagina. The most distal point of anterior wall (point Ba), vaginal cuff scar (point C), and the most distal point of the posterior wall (point Bp) are all at same position (+8), and points Aa and Ap are maximally distal (both at +3). Because TVL equals maximum protrusion, this is stage IV prolapse. (B) Normal support. Points Aa and Ba and points Ap and Bp are all −3 because there is no anterior or posterior wall descent. Lowest point of the cervix is 8 cm above hymen (−8) and posterior fornix is 2 cm above this (−10). Vaginal length is 10 cm and genital hiatus and perineal body measure 2 and 3 cm, respectively. This represents stage 0 support. (*From* Bump RC, Mattiasson A, Bø K, et al. The standardization of terminology of female pelvic organ prolapse and pelvic floor dysfunction. Am J Obstet Gynecol 1996;175(1):14; with permission.)

prolapse may also have urge symptoms and describe symptoms of incomplete emptying. Furthermore, if a patient describes that they used to have stress incontinence but now do not have leakage with stress, they will more likely have a prolapse because sometimes the prolapse will cause a kink of the urethra, stabilizing it so it is less likely to allow for urinary leakage.

For the physical portion of the evaluation, a complete physical is performed. The abdominal examination is especially important because it will be used to evaluate for masses and concurrent pathologic conditions, and will allow for visualization of previous abdominal surgery scars. Patients are placed in the dorsal lithotomy position for the pelvic examination. First, a screening neurologic examination of the motor and sensory areas of the lower extremities and the perineum is performed. Next, a thorough inspection of the labia majora and minora, and surrounding skin, are examined. The urethral meatus and urethra are examined for masses or diverticula. A speculum examination is performed for the condition of the vagina and any lesions, masses, or nonphysiologic discharge. A bimanual examination is performed for and concomitant pathologic conditions with the presentation of prolapse. Next, a POP-Q examination is helpful to objectively evaluate the genital hiatus, perineal body, anterior and posterior vagina, the TVL, and the apex of the vagina.

Office Management

Once prolapse has been diagnosed, patients may be offered multiple types of management. Prolapse is a distressing and uncomfortable condition but it is not life-threatening. It is reasonable to offer conservative management including watching and waiting. Once prolapse is diagnosed, it is often considered a progressive disease, but it is possible it may stay at the same stage or even regress over time.[13] Pelvic floor PT may be offered to decrease symptoms in patients who have POP. A prospective randomized controlled trial found that 19% of patients will decrease the severity of prolapse by 1 stage when undergoing pelvic floor PT.[14] Pelvic floor PT is a minimally invasive way to treat prolapse symptoms; however, it usually requires multiple visits and patients have to continue exercises and the therapy. Sometimes PT will involve placing manometers in the vagina or internal examinations during the treatment and this can be distressing to some patients.

An additional conservative measure for prolapse treatment is the use of vaginal pessaries. Pessaries are medical-grade silicone, rubber, or latex supports that are placed in the vagina to replace the pelvic organs that are prolapsing. Pessaries are ideal for patients who do not want surgery for prolapse or who are not good surgical candidates. They can also be used as temporary relief until the patient is ready for surgery or as a trial to see if the patient's symptoms are indeed from a prolapse. There are 2 main types of pessaries: support and space-occupying. Contraindications for pessary use include allergies to the pessary materials, lesions, or malignancies in the vagina, vaginal infections, or problems with patient compliance. Although many patients can replace and remove their own pessary, some require every follow-up 3 to 6 months. Pessaries neglected and not periodically removed and cleaned can cause erosions, incarceration, or fistulas. Pessaries are often well-tolerated and patients can use them indefinitely, as long as they continue pessary maintenance (**Fig. 5**).

Support Pessaries

Support pessaries can be used for every stage of prolapse. They can be placed and removed by the patient, if needed. They are usually in ring or ovoid forms and may have a diaphragm for extra support. Some examples of support pessaries include rings, rings with support, Gehrungs, continence dishes and pessaries, and Shatz (see **Fig. 5**). Support pessaries are placed in the vagina and held in place by the pubic symphysis, the vaginal introitus, the apex of the vagina, the cervix or uterus, and the pelvic floor muscles. Support pessaries allow for intercourse without removal.

Space-Occupying Pessaries

Space-occupying pessaries tend to be used for more severe staged prolapse (III-IV). They are 3 dimensional and are usually not able to be removed by the patient, so they require regular follow-up at the urogynecology office. Examples of space-occupying pessaries are Gelhorns, cubes, and donuts.

SURGICAL MANAGEMENT

There are multiple surgical options for prolapse. Surgical planning depends on

- Anatomic defects of prolapse
- The general health of the patient
- Patient desire for sexual activity (or not)
- Patient surgical history, including prior prolapse repair
- Patient desires for native tissue repair versus graft-augmented repair

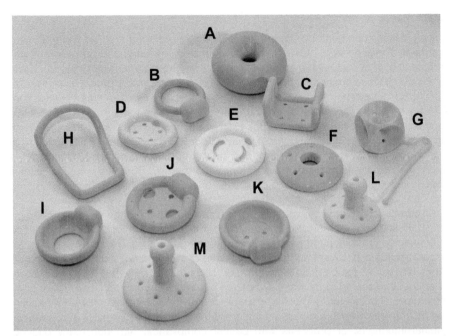

Fig. 5. Types of pessaries. (A) Donut (space-occupying). (B) Ring with knob (continence and support). (C) Gehrung malleable (support). (D) Oval ring with support. (E) Ring with support. (F) Shatz (support). (G) Cube (space-occupying). (H) Hodge (support). (I) Continence dish. (J) Ring with knob with support (support and continence). (K) Continence dish with support (support and continence). (L, M) Gelhorns (space-occupying).

- Concomitant stress incontinence with prolapse
- Patient preference on route of surgery
- Patient lifestyle (eg, daily heavy lifting and exercise).

Anterior prolapse is the most common type of prolapse that presents in patients who will go on to have surgical intervention.[15,16] Repair of the anterior wall may include native tissue repairs, mesh-enhanced repairs and biologic grafts. Anterior wall prolapse is strongly associated with apical prolapse, so when repairing anterior wall defects, often the apex must also be repaired.[17] Apical prolapse can involve a host of techniques, with vaginal approaches or abdominal approaches with laparoscopic or robotic-assistant that may utilize native tissue or synthetic graft material. The repairs may be intraperitoneal or extraperitoneal approaches. The uterosacral ligament suspension allows the vagina to be restored to a more anatomically correct position, however, limited data are available to discern if this is clinically relevant.[18] The gold standard surgery for apical prolapse is the sacrocolpoexy.[19] It anchors the anterior, posterior, and apical compartment of the vagina using synthetic mesh to the anterior longitudinal ligament on the sacrum at S1. Isolated posterior compartment prolapse may be repaired via a transvaginal approach, in which an incision is made in the vagina and the muscularis is reapproximated. Using synthetic mesh or biologic agents have not been found to be beneficial for repair. This procedure is usually performed concomitantly with a perineorrhaphy. Finally, obliterative techniques are used for prolapse to obliterate the vagina, which decreases the chance of recurrent prolapse dramatically. There are 2 approaches. The Le Fort colpocleisis leaves the uterus in place, channels are created on either side of the vagina to allow for discharge from the uterus, and the vagina is then greatly attenuated. A colpocleisis is performed when there is no uterus or at the time of hysterectomy. It includes a vaginectomy, and no channels are created. Colpocleisis is easy and fast, has a high success rate and is a great consideration for patients with concomitant medical problems. However, the patient is not able to have intercourse, and any bleeding cannot adequately be assessed.

SUMMARY

Pelvic organ prolapse and urinary incontinence are common conditions worldwide that may negatively impact a woman's ability to function normally. Fortunately, there are many options to effectively manage these distressing conditions. FPMRS is dedicated to ongoing research centered on prevention and patient outcomes. Although there have not been significant advances in surgical techniques in recent years, vaginal surgery along with technological advances using minimally invasive techniques with laparoscopic and robotic assistance has benefited both patients and surgeons. The authors hope that the future continues to shine light on better options with these life-altering conditions.

Incontinence and pelvic prolapse may be associated with a many factors, such as childbirth, menopause, surgery, and medical conditions. The WPSI states that screening for incontinence across the lifespan is an important component of well-woman health care. Quality of life, physical findings, and mental health all benefit from effective screening and competent stepwise treatment that relies on collaboration between a dedicated team and shared decision-making with patients.

REFERENCES

1. Wu JM, Vaughan CP, Goode PS, et al. Prevalence and trends of symptomatic pelvic floor disorders in U.S. women. Obstet Gynecol 2014;123(1):141–8.
2. Barber MD. Pelvic organ prolapse. BMJ 2016;354.
3. Aoki A, Brown H, Brubaker L, et al. Urinary incontinence in women. Nat Rev Dis Primers 2017;3:17042.
4. Lukacz ES, Whitcomb EL, Lawrence JM, et al. Urinary frequency in community-dwelling women: what is normal? Am J Obstet Gynecol 2009;200:552.
5. Visco AG, Brubaker L, Ritcher HE, et al. Anticholinergic therapy vs OnabotulinumtoxinA for Urgency Urinary Incontinence. N Engl J Med 2012;367(19): 1803–13.
6. Feinberg M. The problems of anticholinergic adverse effects in older patients. Drugs Aging 1993;3(4):335–48.
7. Murray B, Hessami SH, Gultyaev D, et al. Cost-effectiveness of overactive bladder treatments: from the US payer perspective. J Comp Eff Res 2019;8(1): 61–71.
8. Ritcher HE, Burgio KL, Nygaard IE, et al. Continence pessary compared with behavioral therapy or combined therapy for stress incontinence: a randomized control trial. Obstet Gynecol 2010;115(3):609–17.
9. Nager CW, Ritcher HE, Nygaard I, et al. Incontinence pessaries: size, POPQ measures, and successful fitting. Int Urogynecol J 2009;20:1023–8.
10. Haylen BT, Maher CF, Barber MD, et al. An International Urogynecological Association (IUGA)/International Continence Society (ICS) joint report on the terminology for female pelvic organ prolapse (POP). Neurourol Urodyn 2016;27(4): 655–84.

11. Bump RC, Mattiasson A, Bø K, et al. The standardization of terminology of female pelvic organ prolapse and pelvic floor dysfunction. Am J Obstet Gynecol 1996; 175:10.

12. DeLancey JO. Anatomic aspects of vaginal eversion after hysterectomy. Am J Obstet Gynecol 1992;166:1717–24.

13. Handa VL, Garrett E, Hendrix S, et al. Progression and remission of pelvic organ prolapse: a longitudinal study of menopausal women. Am J Obstet Gynecol 2004;190(1):27–32.

14. Braekken IH, Majida M, Engh ME, et al. Can pelvic floor muscle training reverse pelvic organ prolapse and reduce prolapse symptoms? An assessor-blinded, randomized, controlled trial. Am J Obstet Gynecol 2010;203(2):170.e1-7.

15. Barber MD, Maher C. Epidemiology and outcome assessment of pelvic organ prolapse. Int Urogynecol J 2013;24:1783–90.

16. Maher C, Feiner B, Baessler K, et al. Surgery for women with apical vaginal prolapse. Cochrane Database Syst Rev 2016;(11):CD004014.

17. Rooney K, Kenton K, Mueller ER, et al. Advanced anterior vaginal wall prolapse is highly correlated with apical prolapse. Am J Obstet Gynecol 2006;195:1837–40.

18. Barber MD, Brubaker L, Burgio KL, et al. Factorial comparison of two transvaginal surgical approaches and of perioperative behavioral therapy for women with apical vaginal prolapse: the OPTIMAL randomized trial. JAMA 2014;311:1023–34.

19. Maher C, Feiner B, Baessler K, et al. Surgery for women with apical vaginal prolapse. Cochrane Database Syst Rev 2016;(10):CD012376.

Strong Bones, Strong Body

Carolyn J. Crandall, MD, MS, FACP

KEYWORDS

- Fracture • Bone density • Osteoporosis • BMD • DXA
- Dual-energy X-ray absorptiometry

KEY POINTS

- Bone mineral density (BMD) testing should be performed in women 65 years and older.
- For younger women, use a formal risk assessment tool to determine whether BMD testing is recommended.
- Diagnose osteoporosis based on either the occurrence of a hip or vertebral fracture, or a BMD T-score less than or equal to −2.5 by dual-energy x-ray absorptiometry.
- Offer pharmacologic treatment with alendronate, risedronate, zoledronic acid, or denosumab to reduce the risk for hip and vertebral fractures in women who have osteoporosis.
- Treat osteoporotic women with pharmacologic therapy for 5 years. Women at particularly high fracture risk may require longer than 5 years of therapy but optimal duration is unknown. Women who discontinue denosumab should rapidly transition to a bisphosphonate.

INTRODUCTION

Osteoporosis is defined as a systemic skeletal disease characterized by low bone mass and microarchitectural deterioration of bone tissue, with a consequent increase in bone fragility and susceptibility to fracture.[1] Operationally, osteoporosis is diagnosed based on bone mineral density (BMD) measurements (see later discussion) or by the occurrence of fragility fracture.[2,3]

Approximately 4 in 10 white women age 50 years or older will experience a hip, spine, or wrist fracture in the remainder of their lives.[4] The lifetime risk of fracture at age 50 years in the United States is 15% in women.[5] Annual hip fracture rates in the United States are highest in white women (140.7 per 100,000), followed by Asian women (85.4 per 100,000), African American women (57.3 per 100,000), and Hispanic women (49.7 per 100,000).[5] There is similar ethnic and race variability in women for all fractures.[5] Osteoporosis as defined by BMD measurements (T-score ≤−2.5; see later discussion) is less common among non-Hispanic black and Mexican American women than among white women. Nonetheless, in 2010, there were almost 1 million black and Mexican American women aged 50 years and older in the United States with

Dr C.J. Crandall has no conflicts of interest to declare.
Division of General Internal Medicine and Health Services Research, 1100 Glendon Ave., Suite 850-Room 858, Los Angeles, CA 90024, USA
E-mail address: ccrandall@mednet.ucla.edu

BMD in the osteoporosis range, and more than 35 million US women aged 50 years or older had osteoporosis or low bone mass.[6]

The risk of osteoporosis increases with age. Therefore, the aging of the US population carries with it a rapidly increasing potential preventable burden. The number of hip fractures in the United States is expected to double or triple by the year 2040.[7] Each year, the direct medical care costs of osteoporotic fractures in the United States are $17 billion.[8,9] By the year 2025, the numbers of fractures and associated costs in the United States will increase by 50%. The fastest increase is projected to occur in Hispanics, with a 175% increase in the costs of fractures among Hispanics in 2025 compared with 2005.[8]

The consequences of osteoporotic fracture include death, disability, chronic pain, loss of independence, and decreased quality of life. One in 5 women die within 1 year after experiencing a hip fracture.[10] Nearly 40% of people who experience hip fracture are unable to walk independently 1 year following the fracture, and 60% require assistance with at least 1 essential activity of daily living.[11] Osteoporosis is asymptomatic until the occurrence of fracture. Therefore, osteoporosis screening is aimed at the detection and treatment of osteoporosis before the occurrence of a fracture.

SCREENING: WHEN SHOULD SCREENING BEGIN?

Screening is aimed at detecting disease risk or disease at an early stage in large numbers of asymptomatic individuals; in contrast, case-finding is aimed at identifying individuals who are already suspected to be at risk for a disease and/or have signs or symptoms of disease. An example of case-finding in the context of osteoporosis would be BMD testing in persons taking glucocorticoid medications over a prolonged period of time.

The US Preventive Services Task Force (USPSTF) recommends screening for BMD testing in women 65 years and older.[12] The Women's Preventive Services Initiative states that osteoporosis screening should begin at age 65 years, or earlier based on risk factors such as parental history of a hip fracture, smoking, white race, excess alcohol consumption, and low body weight. Such risk factors are part of essential screening tools that assure timely and appropriate screening takes place. To determine which postmenopausal women younger than 65 years are at increased risk of osteoporosis, the USPSTF recommends the use of a formal risk assessment tool (Fig. 1).[12]

Several tools are available to assess osteoporosis risk and are included in the USPSTF guideline (Table 1).[12] These tools seem to perform similarly and are moderately accurate at predicting osteoporosis.[12]

Of the tools listed in the USPSTF osteoporosis screening guideline, the Osteoporosis Self-Assessment Tool (OST) is clearly the simplest to use and is based solely on weight and age (Box 1).[13]

A few studies have been published regarding the use of OST in women aged younger than 65 years. In a study of women in Belgium, the sensitivity of an OST score less than or equal to 1 for identifying women aged 45 to 64 years who had a femoral neck BMD T-score less than or equal to −2.5 was 89%, and specificity was 45%.[14] In the large Women's Health Initiative study of women aged 50 to 64 years at 40 US clinical centers, an OST score less than 2 had a sensitivity of 79%, a specificity of 70%, and a positive predictive value of 15% for identifying femoral neck BMD T-score less than or equal to −2.5.[15] Two smaller single-center studies among women aged 50 to 64 years reported a sensitivities of 56% and 79%, specificities of 69% and 56%, and

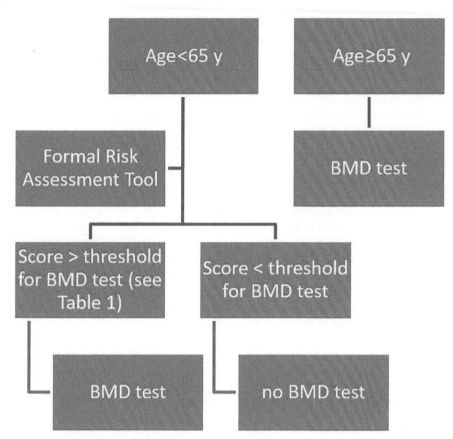

Fig. 1. Recommended use of BMD testing to screen for osteoporosis.

positive predictive values of 35% and 14% using an OST score less than 2 to identify BMD T-score less than or equal to −2.5 at the hip or lumbar spine.[16,17] Therefore, OST has high sensitivity in identifying postmenopausal women with BMD T-score less than or equal to −2.5 (who are candidates for osteoporosis pharmacotherapy). The tools recommended in the USPSTF screening guidelines for selecting women younger than 65 years for BMD testing were selected based on their ability to identify women with BMD T-score less than or equal to −2.5. None of the tools (OST score <2, Simple Calculated Osteoporosis Risk Estimation score >7, Fracture Risk Assessment Tool score ≥9.3%) have high sensitivity for identifying which younger postmenopausal women will experience major osteoporotic fracture during 10 years of follow-up.[18]

SCREENING: WHICH TEST SHOULD BE USED?

Dual-energy X-ray absorptiometry (DXA) is the current gold standard test for diagnosing osteoporosis (in the absence of previous osteoporotic fracture).[2,3]

SCREENING: HOW OFTEN TO PERFORM DUAL-ENERGY X-RAY ABSORPTIOMETRY MEASUREMENT

The optimal frequency of serial BMD testing in the screening setting is unknown. The current evidence does not support frequent monitoring of women with normal BMD for

Table 1
Formal risk osteoporosis assessment tools and commonly used thresholds

Tool	Frequently Used Threshold for Increased Osteoporosis Risk
Osteoporosis Self-Assessment Tool (OST) https://reference.medscape.com/calculator/osteoporosis-self-assessment-women	<2
The Simple Calculated Osteoporosis Risk Estimation (SCORE) https://reference.medscape.com/calculator/osteoporosis-risk-score	≥6
Fracture Risk Assessment Tool (FRAX) https://www.sheffield.ac.uk/FRAX/	≥9.3%[a]
Osteoporosis Index of Risk (OSIRIS)	<1
Osteoporosis Risk Assessment Instrument (ORAI). http://depts.washington.edu/osteoed/tools.php?type=orai	≥9

[a] 9.3% represents the 10-y major osteoporotic fracture risk in a 65-y-old white woman without any other risk factors in the United States, as calculated in 2011. Currently, FRAX calculates this risk to be 8.4%.

Adapted from US Preventive Services Task Force, Curry SJ, Krist AH, et al. Screening for osteoporosis to prevent fractures: US preventive services task force recommendation statement. JAMA 2018;319(24):2526.

osteoporosis because data showed that most women with normal DXA scores did not progress to osteoporosis within 15 years.[2] Hence, the American College of Physicians (ACP) discourages frequent repeated measurements of BMD in women with normal BMD.[2]

The USPSTF guideline[12] states that several observational and modeling studies have suggested that appropriate screening intervals likely depends on age, baseline BMD, and calculated projected time to transition to osteoporosis.[19–21] The USPSTF also points out that 2 good-quality studies found no benefit in predicting fractures from repeating bone measurement testing 4 years[22] to 8 years[23] after initial screening.

SCREENING: WHEN TO STOP BONE MINERAL DENSITY TESTING

The USPSTF screening guidelines do not mention an upper age limit for BMD testing. However, when making decisions about ordering BMD testing, clinicians should recognize that risks versus benefits of osteoporosis pharmacotherapy have not been firmly established in the oldest women (≥80 years old). Also, the benefits versus harms of drug treatment beginning at age 50 to 64 years and continuing over the next

Box 1
Osteoporosis self-assessment tool formula

OST = (weight [kg] − age [years]) × 0.2

Truncate to integer

Adapted from Gourlay ML, Powers JM, Lui LY, et al. Clinical performance of osteoporosis risk assessment tools in women aged 67 years and older. Osteoporos Int 2008;19(8):1175–1183; with permission.

3 decades of life are unknown. If young postmenopausal women use drug treatment, they may have fewer options for pharmacotherapy in their eighth decade of life, when hip fracture risk accelerates.

DIAGNOSIS OF OSTEOPOROSIS USING DUAL-ENERGY X-RAY ABSORPTIOMETRY MEASUREMENTS

Osteoporosis is diagnosed in women aged 50 years and older based on a DXA BMD T-score that lies 2.5 standard deviations or more below the average value for young healthy women; that is, a T-score less than or equal to −2.5 (**Table 2**).[3,24] The recommended reference range is the National Health and Nutrition Examination Survey III reference database for femoral neck measurements in women aged 20 to 29 years.[3] However, the lumbar spine and total hip can also be used for diagnosis in clinical practice.[3] It is of great importance for clinicians to recognize that there are not separate diagnoses for different regions (eg, osteopenia at the hip and osteoporosis at the spine).[24] Among the BMD T-scores of the femoral neck, total hip, and lumbar spine measured by DXA, the diagnosis category is based on the lowest T-score. Guidelines state that each patient receives only a single diagnosis of normal, low BMD, or osteoporosis based on the lowest of the BMD T-scores that were measured by DXA.[24]

LIFESTYLE MEASURES TO OPTIMIZE BONE HEALTH

Strategies for optimizing bone health that are reasonable for clinicians to recommend include avoidance of excessive alcohol use ($\geq$3 units of alcohol daily) and cigarette smoking, and discontinuation of medications that decrease BMD or increase fracture risk, whenever possible. Unfortunately, evidence is insufficient to conclusively show the effect of physical activity on fracture risk.[2] Although data are lacking to determine which type, frequency, and duration of physical activity will reduce fractures, a common clinical practice is to recommend 30 minutes per day of weight-bearing (against gravity) exercise (eg, walking) and gentle resistance exercise a few times per week.

The recommended daily allowance for women aged 31 to 50 years should be 1,000 mg/day of calcium and 600 IU/day of vitamin D. The recommended daily allowance for women aged 51 to 79 years should be 1,200 mg/day for calcium and 600 IU/d of vitamin D. The recommended daily allowance for women aged >/= 70 years should be 1,200 mg/d of calcium and 800 IU/d of vitamin D.

Table 2
Diagnostic classification of bone mineral density results by dual-energy X-ray absorptiometry

Classification	T-Score
Normal	T-score at −1.0 and above
Low bone mass (previously called osteopenia)	T-score between −1.0 and −2.5
Osteoporosis	T-score at or below −2.5
Severe or established osteoporosis	T-score at or below −2.5 with 1 or more fractures

Data from World Health Organization Scientific Group. Assessment of osteoporosis at the primary health care level. Summary report of a WHO Scientific Group. University of Sheffield, Medical School, UK: World Health Organization Collaborating Centre for Metabolic Bone Diseases ;2007; and 2015 ISCD Official Positions – Adult. The International Society for Clinical Densitometry. Available at: https://www.iscd.org/official-positions/2015-iscd-official-positions-adult/. Accessed Oct 11 2018.

The optimal role of calcium and/or vitamin D supplements is controversial. For primary fracture prevention; that is, to prevent fractures among postmenopausal women without osteoporosis or previous fracture, the USPSTF recommends against the use of less than or equal to 400 IU of vitamin D and less than or equal to 1000 mg calcium.[26] The USPSTF also found that evidence is insufficient to recommend greater than 400 IU of vitamin D and greater than 1000 mg calcium in postmenopausal women without osteoporosis or previous fracture.[26] The ACP also concluded that moderate-quality evidence showed that the overall effect of calcium or vitamin D alone on fracture risk is uncertain.[2]

It is important for clinicians to be aware that current evidence is insufficient to assess the balance of benefits and harms of screening for vitamin D deficiency in asymptomatic adults.[27] The benefits of widespread screening for vitamin D deficiency in asymptomatic adults is not supported by current evidence. Instead, clinicians should focus on ensuring that all persons, including those with osteoporosis, receive the recommended daily allowance of calcium and vitamin D intake as laid out by the Institute of Medicine.[25]

The American Society for Preventive Cardiology and the National Osteoporosis Foundation[28] states that

- Obtaining calcium from food sources is preferred.
- Supplemental calcium can be safely used to correct any shortfalls in intake.
- Calcium intake from food and supplements that does not exceed the tolerable upper level of intake (defined by the National Academy of Medicine as 2000–2500 mg/d) should be considered safe from a cardiovascular standpoint.

TREATMENT: WHOM TO TREAT WITH OSTEOPOROSIS PHARMACOTHERAPY AND WITH WHICH MEDICATION

Numerous clinical trials demonstrate that drug therapies reduce fractures in postmenopausal women with osteoporosis. The ACP recommends that alendronate, risedronate, zoledronic acid, or denosumab should be used in women with known osteoporosis. Bisphosphonate treatment should be prescribed for 5 years, but when denosumab is discontinued, rebound fractures may occur. Therefore, if denosumab is discontinued, it should be replaced with another agent, such as a bisphosphonate. The ACP recommends that osteopenic women 65 years of age and older who are at high risk for fracture should be treated based on a discussion of patient preferences, fracture risk profile, and benefits, harms, and costs of medications. The ACP recommends against the use of menopausal estrogen therapy or menopausal estrogen plus progestogen therapy or raloxifene to treatment osteoporosis in women. The ACP recommends against performing bone density monitoring during the 5-year bisphosphonate treatment period for osteoporosis in women.[2,29,30]

Whether and how to treat women with low BMD (osteopenia, BMD T-score between −1 and −2.5) is unclear. The rate of progressive bone loss and the risk for fracture range widely across the osteopenic spectrum and according to additional factors, such as age and the risk for severe adverse events, increases with prolonged use of bisphosphonates.[2] Given limited evidence supporting benefit, the balance of benefits and harms of treating osteopenic women is most favorable when risk for fracture is high.[2] Women younger than 65 years with osteopenia and women older than 65 years with mild osteopenia (T-score between −1.0 and −1.5) will benefit less than women 65 years of age or older with severe osteopenia (T-score <−2.0).[2] In a clinical trial of women with low BMD (T-score >−2.5) but without previous vertebral fractures, 4 years of alendronate did not reduce the risk of clinical fractures.[31]

Recently, after the release of the ACP treatment guidelines, the results of the first randomized controlled trial (RCT) of pharmacotherapy to reduce fracture risk in women with osteopenia aged were published.[32] The trial was a 6-year double-blind RCT of 2000 women 65 years and older with T-scores −1.0 to −2.5 at total hip or femoral neck. The trial compared 4 infusions of zoledronic acid 5 mg or placebo at 18-month intervals. A dietary calcium intake of 1 g/d was advised. Participants who were not already taking vitamin D supplements received cholecalciferol before the trial (single dose of 2.5 mg) and during the trial (1.25 mg/mo). Compared with the placebo group, the zoledronic acid group had nearly a 40% reduction in relative risk for fragility fracture (relative risk 0.63, 95% confidence interval 0.50–0.79). Hip fractures were not a primary endpoint of the trial.

PHARMACOLOGIC TREATMENT DURATION

The ACP recommends that clinicians treat osteoporotic women with pharmacologic therapy for 5 years. However, the ACP acknowledges that appropriate duration of treatment is uncertain and high-risk patients may benefit from greater than 5 years of treatment. Post hoc analysis from an RCT suggested that patients treated with alendronate who had preexisting fractures or those with a BMD of −2.5 or less after 5 years of initial therapy may benefit from continued treatment (10 years total) because these patients experienced a decreased incidence of new clinical vertebral fracture.[2]

After the ACP treatment guideline, new trial results emerged regarding denosumab discontinuation.[33] In a trial of postmenopausal women aged 60 to 90 years with a BMD T-score less than −2.5 at the lumbar spine or total hip, participants received greater than or equal to 2 doses of denosumab or placebo every 6 months, discontinued treatment, and stayed in the study 7 months or longer after last dose. The vertebral fracture rate increased from 1.2 per 100 participant-years during the on-treatment period to 7.1 per 100 participant-years, similar to participants who received and then discontinued placebo (8.5 per 100 participant-years). Most participants (61%) who sustained a vertebral fracture after discontinuing denosumab had multiple vertebral fractures. The investigators concluded that patients who discontinue denosumab should rapidly transition to an alternative antiresorptive treatment.[33]

MONITORING OF BONE MINERAL DENSITY DURING OSTEOPOROSIS PHARMACOTHERAPY

There is no evidence from RCTs regarding how often to monitor BMD during osteoporosis treatment.[2] The ACP recommends against BMD monitoring during the 5-year pharmacologic treatment period for osteoporosis in women.[2] It is critical for clinicians to keep in mind that changes in BMD of less than 3% to 6% at hip and 2% to 4% at the lumbar spine from test to test may be due to the precision error of the test itself. Consequently, guidelines state that DXA reports should contain a statement regarding whether the percent change over time was significant beyond the precision error of the test.[24]

ADVERSE EFFECTS OF OSTEOPOROSIS PHARMACOTHERAPY

Bisphosphonates can cause mild upper gastrointestinal symptoms, atypical femoral fractures, and osteonecrosis of the jaw (ONJ). Raloxifene use is associated with thromboembolic events and stroke death. Zoledronic acid can cause a flu-like syndrome with muscle aches that may be treated with acetaminophen or nonsteroidal antiinflammatory medication, in the absence of contraindications. Teriparatide can cause hypercalcemia and hypercalciuria. These adverse effects are reviewed in the ACP guidelines[2] and underlying evidence reviews.[29,30]

The serious adverse events that have received substantial recent attention are ONJ and atypical subtrochanteric and diaphyseal femoral fractures. ONJ is defined as an area of exposed bone in the oral cavity that does not heal within 8 weeks following identification by a health care provider in a patient who has been receiving or has been exposed to a bisphosphonate or denosumab therapy or antiangiogenic agents, and has not had radiation therapy in the craniofacial region or evidence of local malignancy.[34] ONJ is diagnosed by a dentist or oral surgeon. A recent International Task Force issued recommendations regarding ONJ associated with the use of antiresorptives (bisphosphonates, denosumab) (**Box 2**).[34] The report offers patient educational material regarding ONJ for clinicians to use as handouts.

Routine dental work, such as dental cleaning, fillings, or root canals should be performed as usual and do not require stopping osteoporosis treatment. If major invasive surgery will occur (ie, not simple forceps extraction), then the Task Force recommends that antiresorptive therapy be stopped and restart after mucosal healing (usually 1–2 months).[34] However, there is currently no evidence that interruption of drug therapy in patients requiring dental procedures reduces the risk of ONJ or the progression of the disease.[34]

Atypical subtrochanteric and diaphyseal femoral fractures are the topic of a report of a Task Force of the American Society for Bone and Mineral Research (**Box 3**).[35]

Box 2
Antiresorptive therapy-associated osteonecrosis of the jaw

Risk with low-dose bisphosphonate or denosumab treatment in osteoporosis patients is between 1 in 10,000 and 1 in 100,000 per year, which is increased only slightly, if at all, compared with the risk in the general population who have not taken any osteoporosis therapy.

Risk of ONJ in oncology patients receiving oncology doses of bisphosphonate or denosumab is 1% to 15%

Persons using these medications should see a dentist every 6 months, or as recommended.

Routine dental work, such as dental cleaning, fillings, or root canals should be performed as usual and do not require stopping osteoporosis treatment.

If oral surgery is needed, ideally complete the surgery before starting low-dose oral or yearly intravenous bisphosphonate therapy or denosumab.

Periodontal disease should be managed before starting oncology doses of bisphosphonate or denosumab.

ONJ usually heals with appropriate treatment.

Risk factors for ONJ include major invasive oral surgery, diabetes, glucocorticoid therapy, periodontal disease, denture use, tobacco use, antiangiogenic agents, chemotherapy, radiation therapy, and renal dialysis.

Data from Khan AA, Morrison A, Kendler DL, et al. Case-based review of Osteonecrosis of the Jaw (ONJ) and application of the international recommendations for management from the international task force on ONJ. J Clin Densitom 2017;20(1):8–24.

Box 3
Atypical subtrochanteric and diaphyseal femoral fractures key points
Reported in patients taking bisphosphonates or denosumab
Also occurs in patients with no exposure to these drugs
Absolute risk with bisphosphonates is low: 3.2 to 50 cases per 100,000 person-years
Long-term use may be associated with higher risk ($\sim$100 per 100,000 person-years for 8–9 years use)
Order MRI if there are unilateral or bilateral prodromal symptoms such as dull or aching pain in the groin or thigh
Data from Shane E, Burr D, Abrahamsen B, et al. Atypical subtrochanteric and diaphyseal femoral fractures: second report of a task force of the American Society for Bone and Mineral Research. J Bone Miner Res 2014;29(1):1–23.

SUMMARY

Because osteoporosis is asymptomatic until the occurrence of a fracture, osteoporosis screening is aimed at the detection and treatment of osteoporosis before the occurrence of a fracture. Women aged 65 years or older should receive BMD testing to screen for osteoporosis. Postmenopausal women younger than age 65 years should be screened selectively. BMD testing is recommended for postmenopausal women younger than 65 years at increased risk for osteoporosis, as determined by a formal clinical risk assessment tool. Many formal risk assessment tools are available. The OST tool is the simplest (based on age and weight); it is reasonable to use an OST threshold less than 2 to select candidates for BMD testing among postmenopausal women younger than 65 years old. The optimal frequency of screening is unknown but is strongly influenced by baseline age, baseline BMD value, and the precision error of the machine. Women with normal BMD are unlikely to benefit from frequent rescreening before age 65 years. It is very important for clinicians who order BMD tests to be aware that changes in BMD over time in an individual can only be determined if BMD measurements are made on the same machine. Changes in BMD from test to test over time can be due solely to the precision error of the machine. Guidelines call for the precision error (or least significant change) to be included on DXA reports to aid clinicians in determining whether a significant change has occurred over time.

Guidelines recommend osteoporosis pharmacotherapy for women aged 50 years and older who meet any of the following criteria: (1) BMD T-score less than or equal to −2.5, (2) hip fracture, or (3) vertebral fracture. To decrease hip fracture risk in women, use alendronate, risedronate, zoledronic acid, or denosumab. Teriparatide, raloxifene, and abaloparatide have not been demonstrated to reduce hip fracture risk. The optimal duration of therapy for osteoporosis is unknown. The ACP guidelines recommend 5 years duration of therapy based on existing trial data but acknowledge that some individuals at high risk of fracture may benefit from treatment duration longer than 5 years. Clinical trial data are lacking to inform risks versus benefits of prolonged therapy.

No clinical trials have demonstrated fracture reduction from osteoporosis pharmacotherapy among postmenopausal women younger than age 65 years who have a BMD T-score between −1 and −2.5; thus, these women should be treated selectively based on presence of other fracture risk factors. Scant evidence exists for women aged 65 years or older who have BMD T-score between −1 and −2.5; a single trial showed reduction in fragility fracture, but not specifically hip fracture, with zoledronic acid infusion versus placebo.

Treatment gaps for osteoporosis are significant in the United States. Only 20% of persons who experience hip fracture receive osteoporosis pharmacotherapy within 12 months after discharge.[36,37] Secondary prevention; that is, the targeting of persons with existing fractures for pharmacotherapy to prevent future fracture, is of great importance. Postmenopausal women with hip fracture or vertebral fracture, including those with vertebral fracture detected incidentally, are candidates for osteoporosis pharmacotherapy.

Harms of drug therapies for osteoporosis depend on the specific medication used. The risk of serious adverse events associated with the most common class of osteoporosis medication (bisphosphonates) is no greater than small.

Several important knowledge gaps exist in osteoporosis. Research is needed to address the optimal duration of osteoporosis pharmacotherapy; the role of drug holidays (temporary cessation of osteoporosis pharmacotherapy); the optimal exercise type, intensity, duration, and frequency; the optimal treatment of low bone density (BMD T-score between -1 and -2.5); how to assess bone strength in clinical practice; how to assess fracture risk during pharmacotherapy; and the optimal role of assessment tools for fracture risk in clinical practice.

REFERENCES

1. Consensus development conference: diagnosis, prophylaxis, and treatment of osteoporosis. Am J Med 1993;94(6):646–50.

2. Qaseem A, Forciea MA, McLean RM, et al, Clinical Guidelines Committee of the American College of Physicians. Treatment of low bone density or osteoporosis to prevent fractures in men and women: a clinical practice guideline update from the American College of Physicians. Ann Intern Med 2017;166(11):818–39.

3. World Health Organization Scientific Group. Assessment of osteoporosis at the primary health care level. Summary report of a WHO Scientific Group. University of Sheffield, Medical School, UK. World Health Organization Collaborating Centre for Metabolic Bone Diseases; 2007.

4. U.S. Public Health Service. Bone health and osteoporosis: a report of the surgeon general. Washington, DC: U.S. Dept. of Health and Human Services, Public Health Service, Office of the Surgeon General; 2004. Available at: http://www.surgeongeneral.gov/library.

5. Cauley JA. Defining ethnic and racial differences in osteoporosis and fragility fractures. Clin Orthop Relat Res 2011;469(7):1891–9.

6. Wright NC, Looker AC, Saag KG, et al. The recent prevalence of osteoporosis and low bone mass in the United States based on bone mineral density at the femoral neck or lumbar spine. J Bone Miner Res 2014;29(11):2520–6.

7. Schneider EL, Guralnik JM. The aging of America. Impact on health care costs. JAMA 1990;263(17):2335–40.

8. Burge R, Dawson-Hughes B, Solomon DH, et al. Incidence and economic burden of osteoporosis-related fractures in the United States, 2005-2025. J Bone Miner Res 2007;22(3):465–75.

9. Blume SW, Curtis JR. Medical costs of osteoporosis in the elderly Medicare population. Osteoporos Int 2011;22(6):1835–44.

10. Brauer CA, Coca-Perraillon M, Cutler DM, et al. Incidence and mortality of hip fractures in the United States. JAMA 2009;302(14):1573–9.

11. U.S. Congress OoTA. Hip fracture outcomes in people age 50 and over-background paper. Washington, DC: U.S. Congress Office of Technology Assessment; 1994.

12. US Preventive Services Task Force, Curry SJ, Krist AH, Owens DK, et al. Screening for osteoporosis to prevent fractures: US Preventive Services Task Force recommendation statement. JAMA 2018;319(24):2521–31.

13. Gourlay ML, Powers JM, Lui LY, et al, Study of Osteoporotic Fractures Research Group. Clinical performance of osteoporosis risk assessment tools in women aged 67 years and older. Osteoporos Int 2008;19(8):1175–83.

14. Gourlay ML, Miller WC, Richy F, et al. Performance of osteoporosis risk assessment tools in postmenopausal women aged 45-64 years. Osteoporos Int 2005; 16(8):921–7.

15. Crandall CJ, Larson J, Gourlay ML, et al. Osteoporosis screening in postmenopausal women 50 to 64 years old: comparison of US Preventive Services Task Force strategy and two traditional strategies in the Women's Health Initiative. J Bone Miner Res 2014;29(7):1661–6.

16. Pecina JL, Romanovsky L, Merry SP, et al. Comparison of clinical risk tools for predicting osteoporosis in women ages 50-64. J Am Board Fam Med 2016; 29(2):233–9.

17. Jiang X, Good LE, Spinka R, et al. Osteoporosis screening in postmenopausal women aged 50-64 years: BMI alone compared with current screening tools. Maturitas 2016;83:59–64.

18. Crandall CJ, Larson JC, Watts NB, et al. Comparison of fracture risk prediction by the US Preventive Services Task Force strategy and two alternative strategies in women 50-64 years old in the Women's Health Initiative. J Clin Endocrinol Metab 2014;99(12):4514–22.

19. Gourlay ML, Fine JP, Preisser JS, et al. Bone-density testing interval and transition to osteoporosis in older women. N Engl J Med 2012;366(3):225–33.

20. Gourlay ML, Overman RA, Fine JP, et al. Baseline age and time to major fracture in younger postmenopausal women. Menopause 2015;22(6):589–97.

21. Frost SA, Nguyen ND, Center JR, et al. Timing of repeat BMD measurements: development of an absolute risk-based prognostic model. J Bone Miner Res 2009;24(11):1800–7.

22. Hillier TA, Stone KL, Bauer DC, et al. Evaluating the value of repeat bone mineral density measurement and prediction of fractures in older women: the study of osteoporotic fractures. Arch Intern Med 2007;167(2):155–60.

23. Berry SD, Samelson EJ, Pencina MJ, et al. Repeat bone mineral density screening and prediction of hip and major osteoporotic fracture. JAMA 2013; 310(12):1256–62.

24. 2015 ISCD Official Positions – Adult,. International Society for Clinical Densitometry. Available at: https://www.iscd.org/official-positions/2015-iscd-official-positions-adult/. Accessed October 11, 2018.

25. Institute of Medicine (US) Committee to Review Dietary Reference Intakes for Vitamin D and Calcium, Ross AC, Taylor CL, et al. Dietary reference intakes for calcium and vitamin D. Washington, DC: National Academies Press (US); 2011.

26. US Preventive Services Task Force, Grossman DC, Curry SJ, Owens DK, et al. Vitamin D, calcium, or combined supplementation for the primary prevention of fractures in community-dwelling adults: US Preventive Services Task Force recommendation statement. JAMA 2018;319(15):1592–9.

27. LeFevre ML, US Preventive Services Task Force. Screening for vitamin D deficiency in adults: U.S. Preventive Services Task Force recommendation statement. Ann Intern Med 2015;162(2):133–40.

28. Kopecky SL, Bauer DC, Gulati M, et al. Lack of evidence linking calcium with or without vitamin D supplementation to cardiovascular disease in generally healthy adults: a clinical guideline from the National Osteoporosis Foundation and the American Society for Preventive Cardiology. Ann Intern Med 2016;165(12):867–8.

29. Crandall CJ, Newberry SJ, Diamant A, et al. Comparative effectiveness of pharmacologic treatments to prevent fractures: an updated systematic review. Ann Intern Med 2014;161(10):711–23.

30. Crandall CJ, Newberry SJ, Gellad WG, et al. Treatment to prevent fractures in men and women with low bone density or osteoporosis: Update of a 2007 Report. Comparative Effectiveness Review No. 53. (Prepared by Southern California Evidence-based Practice Center under Contract No. HHSA-290-2007-10062-I). Rockville (MD): Agency for Healthcare Research and Quality; 2012. Available at: www.effectivehealthcare.ahrq.gov/reports/final.cfm.

31. Cummings SR, Black DM, Thompson DE, et al. Effect of alendronate on risk of fracture in women with low bone density but without vertebral fractures: results from the fracture intervention trial. JAMA 1998;280(24):2077–82.

32. Reid I, Horne A, Mihov B, et al. Fracture prevention with zoledronate in older women with osteopenia. N Engl J Med 2018;379(25):2407–16.

33. Cummings SR, Ferrari S, Eastell R, et al. Vertebral fractures after discontinuation of denosumab: a post Hoc analysis of the randomized placebo-controlled FREEDOM trial and its extension. J Bone Miner Res 2018;33(2):190–8.

34. Khan AA, Morrison A, Kendler DL, et al. Case-based review of osteonecrosis of the jaw (ONJ) and application of the international recommendations for management from the International Task Force on ONJ. J Clin Densitom 2017;20(1):8–24.

35. Shane E, Burr D, Abrahamsen B, et al. Atypical subtrochanteric and diaphyseal femoral fractures: second report of a task force of the American Society for Bone and Mineral Research. J Bone Miner Res 2014;29(1):1–23.

36. Solomon DH, Johnston SS, Boytsov NN, et al. Osteoporosis medication use after hip fracture in U.S. patients between 2002 and 2011. J Bone Miner Res 2014; 29(9):1929–37.

37. Gillespie CW, Morin PE. Osteoporosis-related health services utilization following first hip fracture among a cohort of privately-insured women in the United States, 2008-2014: an observational study. J Bone Miner Res 2017;32(5):1052–61.

Section 4: Conclusion

Challenges in the Era of Coding and Corporatization

Mark S. DeFrancesco, MD, MBA[a,b,c,*]

KEYWORDS

- Specialist in obstetrics and gynecology • Population health • Prevention
- Fee-for-service • Value-based care • Primary care • Corporatization of medicine

KEY POINTS

- There have been multiple new challenges to the "annual visit" in recent years.
- There has been an increase in the number of graduates going into subspecialties, reducing the number of Obstetrician-Gynecologists in "general" practice at the same time the increased numbers of subspecialists significantly limit the role of the general Obstetrician-Gynecologist.
- Health care has also changed, with an emphasis shifting from intervention to prevention, and a new focus on population health.
- This is an opportunity for the Obstetrician-Gynecologist to succeed in the new health care field as payment models are shifted from "fee-for-service" to "value-based care."
- Many women still see their women's health care providers as being their "primary" care provider. We must step up and provide the care they deserve.

INTRODUCTION

In the 1970s and earlier, patients made appointments to see a doctor anytime they were ill or had a medical problem arise. Although undoubtedly some patients did schedule a "physical" or "annual" examination, generally no one spoke in terms of "preventive care." An "annual" in women's health care parlance really meant a Papanicolaou (Pap) smear, a breast examination, and a pelvic examination, at least in the Obstetrician-Gynecologist's office. The addition of pharmaceutical contraceptives contributed to more routinized visits to Obstetrician-Gynecologist practices during the ensuing decades.

Many women have long-term relationships with their Obstetrician-Gynecologists, and many Obstetrician-Gynecologists have experienced the satisfaction of providing

Disclosure: No conflicts of interest to disclose.
[a] Department of Obstetrics and Gynecology, University of Connecticut, Farmington, CT, USA;
[b] Women's Health Connecticut, Avon, CT, USA; [c] American College of Obstetricians and Gynecologists, Washington, DC, USA
* 60 Westwood Avenue, Suite 200, Waterbury, CT 06708.
E-mail address: mdefrancesco@womenshealthct.com

Obstet Gynecol Clin N Am 46 (2019) 553–561
https://doi.org/10.1016/j.ogc.2019.04.012
0889-8545/19/© 2019 Elsevier Inc. All rights reserved.

obgyn.theclinics.com

care to 2 or more generations within families. Changes taking place in health care, and in our specialty specifically, raise challenges to current practice. Challenges include, but are not limited to, increasing subspecialization and the changing scope of practice, documentation changes and pressures in the digital world, and the corporatization of medicine with small independent practices disappearing. This article reviews challenges and presents strategies to meet them directly and transform them into opportunities for improvement.

CHALLENGES TO THE "ANNUAL VISIT"

The "annual visit" has long been established as part of women's health care. Most insurers cover the visit without co-pays or deductibles and recognize it as a valuable contact with the health system, worthy of being encouraged. As noted in the introduction of this article, preventive care contributes to women's overall health and wellbeing.

Recent advances in women's health have led to significant pushback from some patients and organizations questioning the need for an annual visit. For instance, the improvements in cervical cancer screening have led to extending the screening interval to 3 to 5 years. However, because the screening recommendations began changing in 2004, no studies are found that report any significant decline in the number of patients returning annually for visits.

Another magnet that long kept patients adherent to an annual routine was the requirement of prescriptions for oral contraceptives. With the advent of long-acting reversible contraception (LARC), the need for an annual prescription is eliminated. Interestingly, there is no reported decline in the number of patients with LARC who return for an annual examination.

The annual examination has been challenged by the misinterpretation of recommendations about the utility of a routine pelvic examination in otherwise asymptomatic women.[1] The annual examination goes well beyond the pelvic examination.

The well-woman examination should not be regarded by patient or physician as simply a "Pap and pelvic examination." Rather, it is an opportunity for a comprehensive contact with the health care system to take advantage of preventive services and thus contribute to a patient's overall wellness. We need to recognize the shift from intervention to prevention.

THE CHALLENGE OF SUBSPECIALIZATION

Today, the scope of women's health care is changing. Consider that in the mid-1980s, when the author of this article finished residency training, it was generally routine practice for most new graduates to go into private practice and provide a full scope of services.

In 2000, only 7% of residency graduates went on for fellowship training, and most of the remainder went into clinical practice, either "private" or university based, without subspecializing.[2] Graduates handled a wide variety of cases, ranging across most of the now "subspecialized" areas of high-risk obstetrics, gynecologic oncology, infertility, and urogynecology. Minimally invasive surgery was limited to tubal fulguration and diagnostic indications, and the laparoscope was the tool of the "general" Obstetrician-Gynecologist for years before it was discovered by the general surgeons and other specialties.

The scope of general obstetrical-gynecologic practice has changed significantly. In 2017, almost 30% of graduates entered fellowship training in the subspecialties.[3]

Many more subspecialists are located in populated areas of the country, and the knowledge base in each of the subspecialty areas has grown geometrically.

For a practice to provide a wide range of services today, the practice must become a "well-rounded" collection of individual providers with focused skill sets as opposed to a collection of "well-rounded" individual providers who can each "do it all." What does this mean for many Obstetrician-Gynecologists who are not subspecialists? For the more senior physicians, it may mean giving up some of the procedures and surgeries they did, and did competently, years ago. There are newer techniques, instruments, and technologies that can better serve our patients, and unless we master the knowledge base pertaining to that subspecialty, and also achieve the volume and outcomes of the subspecialist, the ethical alternative is to refer a patient for that operation or treatment.

Alternatives to major surgery like hysterectomy have emerged, and nonsurgical means of treating heavy bleeding or fibroids play a larger role in our specialty. Office-based procedures have made treatment of patients more accessible and affordable.

Although the scope of general obstetrics and gynecology practice has been influenced by increasing subspecialization and presents a challenge to many providers who wish to practice the full scope of obstetrics and gynecology, we have an opportunity to adapt, which the author discusses later in this article.

THE CHALLENGE OF DOCUMENTATION AND THE ELECTRONIC MEDICAL RECORD

Another major difference between now and the author's very early years in practice is in clinical documentation. Rather than causing physicians to feel like they were performing data entry for insurance companies, office records were crisp and concise and contained pertinent positives and negatives. To be fair, because they were handwritten and stored in the "file room" of a practice, legibility was often a problem as was lack of accessibility when the office was closed. Nevertheless, from a "workflow" point of view, the simplicity of the written medical record had some positive points.

Today, although electronic health records may still hold the promise of making health care more rational, safe, and effective, most systems have a long way to go to achieve those goals. An electronic record offers accessibility, data collection, and proactive patient management, all ideal goals in health care. However, during this interim, disruptive time in health care, electronic medical records (EMRs) are often perceived as contributing heavily to the current "burnout" crisis in health care.[3,4]

That notwithstanding, for the purposes of this article, the EMR discussion is limited. One of the key challenges we face in the digital era of health care is the need to improve electronic documentation to where systems can be interoperable, contain relevant medical decision-making algorithms and meaningful, appropriate red flags and alarms, in order to truly make systems reach their potential to help with the delivery of high-quality and cost-effective care.

The very cost of EMR is often prohibitive, especially for solo and very small group practices.[5] It appears to be one of the main drivers in the decision being made by physicians to either retire earlier than planned, or to transition from a small practice to a larger practice, or to a hospital or health system as an employed physician.

The growth of these larger group practices and health systems has helped pay for these expensive systems. In addition, federally funded programs like HITECH have helped with some of the cost of EMR implementation, but they have not solved the significant EMR-related problems that negatively impact practices because of the time and energy needed for implementation. These issues are workflow issues that are a source of real frustration among clinicians.

The National Academy of Medicine (formerly the Institute of Medicine) has identified EMR-related angst as one of the primary causes of burnout and is addressing it, with its Action Collaborative on Clinician Resilience and Well-Being. It has already developed several important position papers focused on this topic.[6,7]

Most EMRs have evolved from billing systems, and clinical office workflow is being modified significantly but in a Procrustean way to fit such legacy systems. The electronic record has the potential to vastly improve the quality of care, and the ability to create systematic outreach so that all patients receive appropriate preventive health care at the appropriate intervals. Rather than being a hindrance, a properly designed EMR can improve care delivery. There is hope that this problem is starting to resolve as artificial intelligence is developing and may provide "smarter" solutions.

THE CHALLENGE OF CORPORATIZATION

Since 1960, we have seen tremendous growth in the cost of health care in the United States, measured in absolute dollars, as a percent of gross domestic product (GDP) and also as a per-capita cost. For example, in 1960, total dollars spent on health care were tallied at $27 billion, compared with $3.492 trillion spent in 2017. Expressed per capita, the increase went from $146 per capita in 1960 to $10,739 in 2017. As a percent of GDP, it increased from 5% in 1960 to 17.9% in 2017.

That is a large amount of math to digest, but what does it mean for our purposes? The bottom line is that it shows how much more expensive it is to provide health care today than in 1960. As more insurance companies evolved and more people were covered, especially with the start of Medicare and Medicaid in the mid-1960s, costs naturally increased.

Drivers were complex and multifactorial, but they include increased utilization as more people used more services that were now "paid" by the insurer and not directly out of pocket; new pharmaceuticals that were much more expensive, in part to recoup research and development costs, but also, to pursue the profit that came along with the sales of the "next new thing"; significant growth in the insurance industry itself with a need for more middle management people and a host of utilization review and related employees; and, of course, the burgeoning of not only salaries but also golden parachutes for CEOs and very senior management people in insurance companies, hospitals, and health systems.

All of these contribute far more to the cost of health care than do provider salaries. However, when it became apparent that something needed to be done to hold down the cost of health care, it engendered a corporate response. As long ago as 1990, it was recognized that insurers were under great pressure to reorganize health care. This pressure was from the major payers involved: the government and private businesses that were paying the bill for their employees. It was foreseen that "medical management information systems applications" would produce algorithms and protocols that would "constrain wide variations in the practice of medicine" and generally seek to "improve the productivity of physicians." Furthermore, it was also accurately predicted that the "medical profession is likely to be subjected to far more administrative and bureaucratic controls than conceivable even a few years ago."[8]

Well, all this has come to pass. The corporatization of medicine has resulted in part in declining physician income, at least relative to the general upward trend that has characterized staff salaries, office rental costs, insurance costs (health insurance and professional liability insurance), and, of course, the cost of supplies and drugs, during these past 40 years. This reality has created a real pressure on practices to be more "productive" in the sense of seeing more patients in a limited amount of time in order to generate the revenues needed to pay all the expenses of a practice, most of which continued to increase with the tide while the physician's salary remained tethered to the anchor of "managed cost" and antitrust laws that prohibited opportunities for successful rate negotiations, at least for solo and very small practices.

All that being said, our mission in health care is to provide the best care possible for our patients and to advocate for them in an ever-increasing corporate system of care. That is the real challenge of corporatization. It is not about getting paid more for our services, although it often takes strong negotiation to get paid enough to keep the doors open. The real challenge of corporatization is to ensure that utilization rules and regulations dictated by insurers are consistent with high quality health care.

Yes, we need to be cost conscious, but only insofar as that is what will help save the system and keep it operational and providing more care for more people. It should never be to help the insurance company grow profits. Once again, we have hit on a topic that could be the subject of an entire book. Consequently, at this point, consideration of the patient is the next focus.

CHALLENGE TO OUR PATIENTS

Shifting the spotlight a bit illuminates the problems our patients face more with the health care system. They used to see their physician, or what we now call a "primary care provider," as their only doctor, providing most of the care they needed. As more subspecialization and increasing regulation from payers and the government grew, the system has become more difficult to navigate. In addition, many women for many of their younger, "healthier" years only see their Obstetrician-Gynecologist as a health care provider; we need to recognize and respond to the responsibility that places on us.

To do that, we need to provide more comprehensive care to our patients. We must recognize that the patient's blood pressure, weight, smoking status, cardiac health, and many other facets of their well-being are our responsibility, at least during the many years that we are their routine contact with the health care system. In many ways, we may be missing the boat in areas where we could be doing a much better job, if we were just thinking more broadly about "women's health." Being more comprehensive does not mean we must be able to treat complex medical conditions that may arise in our patients, but we should be doing appropriate screening for these conditions and referring them to the specialists who do treat these problems. As Dr Diana E. Ramos introduces in the article, "Preconception Health: Changing the Paradigm on Well-Woman Health," in this issue, the Women's Preventive Services Initiative provides a table that summarizes screenings across a woman's lifespan that should be used to make sure patients receive adequate attention to preventive care.

Even more importantly, we should look for the low-hanging fruit: the easy screenings to find and work on, not requiring complex diagnostic testing to discover. For example, during the course of the years during which Obstetrician-Gynecologists provide care for their patients, many patients who were smokers continued to smoke. There is evidence that many patients do in fact want to stop smoking and need real encouragement to do so.[9] We need to go beyond a simple formulaic suggestion that patients quit tobacco and be more engaged with them with some basic education about health effects and even the economic cost to them of continuing to smoke. Payers would be well advised to start reimbursing practices for follow-up visits to assist the patient.[10]

In a similar vein, it is just as likely that our patients gained significant weight over the years we provided their care. Short term, those extra pounds were not noticeable, but over 30 years they could add up to as much as 40-50 kgs! Up until now, if a patient was a smoker, or weighed too much, most doctors did not say much about either issue. It just was not seen as part of an Obstetrician-Gynecologist practice (with the possible exception of monitoring weight gain during pregnancy), but we were failing our patients.

I think about why we do what we do. Why did we become doctors? We presumably wanted to positively impact the health of our patients, save lives, and help people be healthy. More specifically, why are we in women's health? Many of us were attracted to the field in part by the combination of varied experiences in providing women's health, including but not limited to surgery, delivering babies, and detecting and treating cancer and precancerous conditions. In addition, it is a specialty that establishes long-term relationships with most patients over many years of their lives. That being the case, it should be a natural next step in the evolution of women's health practice to address how we can best impact the lives of our patients, and at the same time, have a positive influence on what is today called population health, the health of our nation.

One of the most direct areas in which we impact the health of our patients is of course in cancer detection and prevention. In our "traditional" Obstetrician-Gynecologist practice, we have made tremendous strides, especially in cervical cancer detection and prevention as well as in helping in the detection of breast and (to a lesser extent perhaps) ovary problems. As Drs Alison Vogell and Megan L. Evans state in the article, "Cancer Screening in Women," in this issue, cancer screening techniques in the past 50 years have allowed for earlier detection of cancer at premalignant or early stages of disease allowing for significant reductions in morbidity and mortality. However, when looking at the total number of deaths in the United States from breast, uterus, ovary, and cervix combined, it is just about 70,000 each year.[11] Consequently, assuming we could improve our success rate to 100%, we could possibly save 70,000 lives each year. That figure is a reasonable potential to do some real good, and we, of course, should not abandon the traditional elements of practice that focus on these areas. However, let us go beyond that.

Look at other issues causing even more deaths annually in the United States. Smoking and obesity are 2 areas that together are responsible for an estimated 780,000 deaths each year, more than 10 times the number of deaths caused by "traditional" gynecologic-related cancers. Smoking alone (including secondhand smoke) leads to 480,000 deaths annually.[12] Obesity is the cause of another 300,000 deaths each year according to a fairly conservative estimate.[13] Clearly, by broadening our scope of practice to include a strong element of prevention, we can potentially save many more lives and maybe even help reverse the worldwide obesity epidemic.

The author would like to repeat the challenge he first issued in 2015, to ask women's health care providers everywhere to include smoking and obesity among the many things we should be addressing with our patients. These areas are 2 areas in which we might make some real progress, if addressed aggressively and continuously in our practice.

This issue of Obstetrics and Gynecology Clinics of North America has summarized the screening goals of The Women's Preventive Services Initiative (WPSI). Depression, intimate partner violence, bone health, bladder function, genetic risks, and environmental exposures, are recognized as essential elements in ongoing comprehensive preventive care. Finding potential problems and preventing them is a much more efficient way to lower costs in health care and improve quality outcomes.

THE CHALLENGE OF "BATTING CLEAN-UP"

It is a real honor to be contributing an article to this issue, and especially, to be writing the summary article in what will certainly be regarded as a seminal work in the continued evolution of women's health care.

It was about 20 years ago that American College of Obstetricians and Gynecologists adopted the subtitle "Women's Health Care Physicians" to broaden the perceived scope of the Obstetrician-Gynecologist. We were starting to recognize that Obstetrics and Gynecology was not just about delivering babies, performing hysterectomies, and doing breast and pelvic examinations. Women's health is more comprehensive, especially as we recognize the importance of gender-specific health concerns that require expertise of a "women's health" provider.

Simultaneously, technology has intervened, and birth rates have dropped and so has the standard "bread-and-butter" business of the traditional Obstetrician-Gynecologist office. There are fewer babies being born; the interval for cervical cancer screening is extended so Pap smears are less frequently needed; LARC has reduced the number of annually renewed oral contraception prescriptions, and the number of hysterectomies is contracting with the increase of endometrial ablation, uterine artery embolization, and progestin-containing intrauterine devices that reduce hemorrhage complaints.

In addition to these observations, the increased number of subspecialists available in all areas (REI, UroGyn, MIGS, GynOnc and MFM) has resulted in moving more cases to tertiary levels for more expert approach for many of the problems that were routinely addressed in the "generalist" office years ago.

The upshot of these changes was that the "specialist in obstetrics and gynecology" (typically referred to as a "generalist") has far less to do, if she or he is referring "complicated" patients to appropriate subspecialists, and of course, if she or he is using newer technology to address issues that previously were addressed surgically. Consequently, how to fill that void? Read on.

RESPONSES TO THE CHALLENGES

We have considered various challenges in the modern era of health care. These challenges include threats to the annual visit, the unintended consequences of increasing subspecialization, the tremendous impact of digital documentation requirements, the corporatization of medicine, and the challenges to our patient's collective health, the health of our nation, and world actually, posed especially by smoking, obesity, and environmental concerns, as voiced by Drs Kelly McCue and Nathaniel DeNicola and in the article, "Environmental Exposures in Reproductive Health," in this issue.

We can address these challenges by reengineering our practices; not necessarily a major makeover, but rational changes to add services and screenings that our patients deserve and that are well within our competence. Our goal would not be to master all areas of medicine, but at the very least, our goal would be to screen selectively as recommended by WPSI. Smoking, obesity, hypertension, hyperlipidemia, thyroid dysfunction, and diabetes are conditions for which we need not provide comprehensive care, but for which screening and referrals are appropriate.

Given the challenges, the shift from a traditional "fee-for-service" payment system to "value-based care" will help address these challenges. Value-based care is a system that will pay health care providers to keep populations of people healthy, measuring good outcomes and adding value to the system. No doubt that may sound a bit Pollyanna-ish, but let me explain.

This is a disruptive time in medicine and in the business of health care. Just as the telephone replaced the telegraph, and the automobile replaced horses and buggies, the next payment model in health care will undoubtedly replace the traditional fee-for-service system. The extent of replacement may vary by specialty, and there may be hybrid systems that modify rather than replace the traditional model, but change will undoubtedly come.

Change will encourage us to broaden the services we offer our patients and to provide the best care that every woman deserves, in a convenient "one-stop shop." This approach will increase value to patients and attract payers who can determine where patients receive care. It will also lead us to realize the value of a health care team to provide that care, where every team member works up to the limits of her or his license. This method can provide more care to more people and increase the quality of care through systematic outreach.

Consequently, the "annual" examination should be modified to include various screenings, as recommended, only at specified intervals. The alternate years provide more time in that visit to address other concerns perhaps also not requiring annual screening. The ideal EMR will help achieve such goal, through a systematic outreach and alert system. The list of recommended screenings and relevant intervals should be integrated into the EMR schedule of annual visits that cover such cycles to ensure that all recommended services are provided in a timely fashion.

This issue covers many of the topics that are relevant to the provision of preventive services for women. In addition, Women's Preventive Services Guidelines can be found at https://www.womenspreventivehealth.org/, and these will be updated on a regular basis as a reference to keep a practice tuned into the most up-to-date recommendations.

THE FINAL CHALLENGE

There is one more challenge we have not yet raised: the challenge to the "soul" of our profession. We must maintain our professionalism in an age where "guild interests" are becoming more dominant and are being perceived as the only way to survive in an increasingly complex world of health care business. In a very timely article, Drs Chervenak, McCullough, and Hale remind us that we should guard against powerful forces that "now exist that could subordinate professionalism to guild self-interest."[14]

That is an extremely important message to never lose sight of in this new world of health care business. The development of large group practices is a fact of life in this new world as well as the absorption of many solo or small practices into hospital-based health systems. Although the "business person" is primarily responsible to shareholders and the production of profits, the "professionals," who *we* are, are responsible to our patients. We pursue "profit" to the extent that it allows our practice to survive and enjoy enough "clout" to advocate for our patients.

There is a long tradition of a firewall between physicians and industry, born of the recognition and acknowledgment of the duty we have to patients and the extraordinary trust they put in us. Many years ago, there was not much interplay between the payer and the physician. The relationship was primarily between the physician and the patient. Gradually, the insurer has engaged the physician more directly, especially as managed care evolved.

The need to deal directly with insurers in part has led to the growth of large provider groups, which began in the mid-1990s but is accelerating even more this past decade.

The development of these large groups can be seen as 1 way to preserve "private practice." It also gives physician members a seat at the table when dealing with insurers. However, all care must be taken to use this power only for good.

Consequently, the challenge to not lose our "soul" as we grow into stronger organizations and gain some leverage at the bargaining table is to do so seeking only better care for patients, not simply better contracted payment rates, but also to pressure payers to work with us to do the right thing for patients when making coverage decisions and build quality programs with payers that will help us move the needle on improving the health care of our nation. This approach relies on physicians placing the quality and delivery of patient care first. That is how we can meet many of the challenges discussed in this article, provide care for our patients and our physicians, and not lose our soul.

REFERENCES

1. Levy B. Is the annual pelvic exam a relic or a requisite? OBG Manag 2011;23(4): 14–20.
2. Rayburn WF. The obstetrician-gynecologist workforce in the United States: facts, figures and implications. Washington, DC: ACOG; 2017. p. 2.
3. Available at: https://www.beckershospitalreview.com/healthcare-information-tech nology/mayo-study-links-ehrs-with-physician-burnout.html. Accessed December 21, 2018.
4. Available at: https://hbr.org/2018/03/to-combat-physician-burnout-and-improve-care-fix-the-electronic-health-record. Accessed December 21, 2018.
5. Available at: https://www.ncbi.nlm.nih.gov/pmc/articles/PMC5089148/. Accessed December 21, 2018.
6. Horvath K, Sengstack P, et al. 2018. A vision for a person-centered health information system. NAM Perspectives. Discussion Paper, National Academy of Medicine. Washington, DC, October 3–5, 2018. Available at: https://doi.org/10.31478/201810a.
7. Ommaya AK, Cipriano PF. 2018. Care-centered clinical documentation in the digital environment: solutions to alleviate burnout. NAM Perspectives. Discussion Paper, National Academy of Medicine. Washington, DC, October 3–5, 2018. https://doi.org/10.31478/201801c.
8. Feinglass J, Salmon JW. Corporatization of medicine: the use of medical management information systems to increase the clinical productivity of physicians [review]. Int J Health Serv 1990;20(2):233–52.
9. Available at: https://www.surgeongeneral.gov/library/reports/50-years-of-progress/full-report.pdf. Accessed December 20, 2018.
10. Available at: https://opmed.doximity.com/articles/our-health-system-is-a-sick-system. Accessed December 28, 2018.
11. Available at: https://www.cancer.org/content/dam/cancer-org/research/cancer-facts-and-statistics/annual-cancer-facts-and-figures/2017/leading-sites-of-new-cancer-cases-and-deaths-2017-estimates.pdf. Accessed December 27, 2018.
12. Available at: https://www.cdc.gov/tobacco/data_statistics/fact_sheets/fast_facts/index.htm. Accessed December 28, 2018.
13. Available at: https://www.wvdhhr.org/bph/oehp/obesity/mortality.htm. Accessed December 28, 2018.
14. Chervenak FA, McCullough LB, Hale RW. Guild interests: an insidious threat to professionalism in obstetrics and gynecology. Am J Obstet Gynecol 2018;219: 581–4.

Printed and bound by CPI Group (UK) Ltd, Croydon, CR0 4YY

03/10/2024

01040406-0018